Susan Saunders is a health coach and author. Through one-to-one coaching, workshops and classes, she helps people across the world power up post-menopause and reduce their dementia risk. She is co-creator of The Age-Well Project platform.

www.susansaundershealth.com

The
How to
Power
thrive after
Decade
Menopause

Susan Saunders

Copyright © 2023 Susan Saunders

The right of Susan Saunders to be identified as the Author of
the Work has been asserted by her in accordance with the
Copyright, Designs and Patents Act 1988.

First published in 2023 by Headline Home
an imprint of Headline Publishing Group

First published in paperback in 2024

1

Cataloguing in Publication Data is available from the British Library

ISBN 978 1 4722 9161 5
e-ISBN 978 1 4722 9162 2

Designed and Typeset by Avon DataSet Ltd, Alcester, Warwickshire

Printed and bound in Great Britain by Clays Ltd, Elcograf S.p.A.

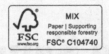

MIX
Paper | Supporting
responsible forestry
FSC® C104740

Headline's policy is to use papers that are natural, renewable and recyclable
products and made from wood grown in well-managed forests and other
controlled sources. The logging and manufacturing processes are expected
to conform to the environmental regulations of the country of origin.

HEADLINE PUBLISHING GROUP
An Hachette UK Company
Carmelite House
50 Victoria Embankment
London EC4Y 0DZ

www.headline.co.uk
www.hachette.co.uk

For Honor and Unity, my power duo

Contents

MIND

SECTION 4: YOU HAVE THE POWER: REDUCE THE RISK OF LONG-TERM HEALTH ISSUES

SECTION 1

YOUR POWER DECADE STARTS HERE

Introduction: Welcome to Your Power Decade

*'There is no greater power in the world
than the zest of a post-menopausal woman'*
MARGARET MEAD (1901–1978), AMERICAN ANTHROPOLOGIST

This book is for you if you're ready to grab some of that zest, power up and face the future head on. Are you excited to build the life you want after fifty, with good health at its heart? This is your time to create the adventures – large and small – you want in your life. The power decade is yours to enjoy if you're past the hormonal rollercoaster of peri-menopause and in your fifties or sixties, ready to prioritise your health, your wellbeing and your future.

Behind us are years that have been spent building a life, a career, a home. Ahead of us – by our mid-sixties – may be retirement, travel, downsizing, possible grandparenthood. In between is a decade or so we've been gifted to create that future. As our physical fertility goes, our creative, mental and emotional fertility ramps up. We're free from the monthly rolling tides of menstruation and ready to reclaim who we really are, untethered from the powerful cycles that dominated our lives for so long.

If we do the maths, we may live half our adult lives post-menopause: there's thirty-three years between reaching adulthood at eighteen and the average age of menopause at fifty-one, and another thirty-two years before we hit the average female life expectancy in the UK of eighty-three.[1] If we look after ourselves, and luck is on our side, we have many years ahead to enjoy the post-menopausal zest that anthropologist Margaret Mead identified. The decade that takes us from our mid-fifties to mid-sixties is a time for us to forge ahead, to decide who we are and how we want to live. And, as a health coach, I know the foundation for this is our own health: physical and mental.

The years immediately after the menopause transition are the most important for a woman's health.* We want to feel our best right now and create a firm foundation for the future. Statistically, the chronic diseases of ageing may take root by the time we reach our mid-sixties. The influential *Lancet* journal described menopause as a turning point for health, saying: 'Many important conditions occur ten to fifteen years after menopause, including weight gain and obesity, metabolic syndrome, diabetes, osteoporosis, arthritis, cardiovascular disease, dementia and cancer; therefore,

---

* I use the term women throughout the book, but I am, of course, referring to all those born with a uterus – women, non-binary and transpeople: anyone who experiences menopause.

the occurrence of menopause heralds an important opportunity to institute preventative strategies.'[2]

That gives us around a decade after the average age we reach menopause (and I know that no one is average and every experience is different) to focus on being in the best health we can. Conscious of both hormone change and ageing, we want to thrive now, and in the future. In this book I coach you through the preventative strategies you need, and make sure you have the right knowledge, mindset and motivation to power up and put them into action.

WHO AM I?

I experienced perimenopause in a daze through my forties, unaware, really, of what was happening to me. I knew I had a cluster of symptoms: erratic periods, crashing mood swings, hot flushes and more. My GP told me everything was normal. Complementary therapies didn't help. No one told me that I was going through a profound shift, in terms of my metabolic, heart, bone and mental health.

Post-menopause, I have felt a tremendous sense of renewal despite seismic life changes: bereavement, an empty nest, a change of career. I felt I was shedding several skins at once. As a result, I continue to work on my health, which includes taking hormone replacement therapy (HRT), and I feel stronger, physically and mentally, than at any other time in my life.

In my late forties I founded The Age-Well Project with my friend Annabel Streets, and we wrote a book of the same name together. We started with the premise that healthy ageing is about taking control, preparing our minds and bodies for what should be the best years of our lives. While we were writing the book, I realised I wanted to do more to help women to age well and made my own midlife career pivot. I qualified as a health coach with the Institute of Integrative Nutrition, then undertook the Institute's advanced coaching qualification. I've also trained as a dementia prevention coach with American neuro-scientist Dr Dale Bredesen, author of *The End of Alzheimer's*, and his team.

Now I coach women to take charge of their health post-menopause, reduce their dementia risk and age well. I've seen tremendous transformations in the hundreds of women I've coached: some of my clients move me to tears with the extraordinary leaps they make. These are women who want to make the best of their health post-menopause, and experience their own power decades. One said to me recently, 'I was on a downward slope until we started work-ing together: you provided the impetus to make changes and made me more accountable for my health. You've steered me onto the right pathway.'

This book is all about finding the right pathway for you.

WHAT IS HEALTH COACHING?

Being a health coach is a privilege: I get to go on a journey with wonderful women who want to make the best of their lives. It's a collaborative process, and they're in the driving seat. I tell my clients to imagine that we're on a tandem bicycle together: I'm in the back providing the power, they're in the front deciding the direction of travel.

I don't dictate a lifestyle to my clients, and I won't to you either. I'll give you the tools and skills you need to improve your own health and wellbeing. And I'll hold you accountable as you go through the process of change. A health coach's superpower is motivating behavioural change: my clients know that I'm there to be the voice in their ear reminding them to prioritise their health. Clients tell me they ask themselves, 'What would Susan do?'!

Let's grab this opportunity for good health together and make the years to come your best yet.

DISCLAIMER

I'm not a doctor or a nurse. I can't prescribe; I can't give you advice on individual health issues. You need to talk to your GP about those. I'm here to guide you to make your own healthy choices, and to coach you to discover what's right for you.

How to Use this Book

This book is designed to give you maximum flexibility: you can start here and keep working through to create a whole lifestyle to support your health post-menopause. Or you can dip into the specific sections most relevant to your concerns. Worried about your stress levels? Turn to page 149 for a detailed breakdown of why they're rising and what to do. Want to know how to eat to maintain bone density? That's on page 217. Know you'd benefit from inspiring stories of other women making the most of their own power decades? You'll find these at the end of each section in our POWER WOMEN profiles.

I've talked to many inspirational women – and brilliant experts – to find out from them how best to power up in the years ahead. You'll find their input throughout the book, particularly so from my three 'wise women', menopause specialists Dr Carys Sonnenberg, Dr Fionnuala Barton and Dr Juliet Balfour.

In the rest of **SECTION 1** you'll find a breakdown of what happens to our bodies during the menopause transition, the symptoms we may have experienced, or are still experiencing, the role of oestrogen and other reproductive hormones in our health, and some thoughts on HRT.

SECTION 2 is all about how to build your power decade – how to claim this time as your own and create a foundation of good health. We dive into what I call the 'three Ms' of the power decade – the key areas to focus on after the 'M' of the menopause transition.

How we think, eat and exercise provides our momentum through this time of change. Get these right and we set the foundations for a healthier and happier ever after. And you know what? None of these are difficult: it's about small daily habits that build up to huge changes. It's often the tiniest lifestyle tweaks that can have the biggest impact.

There are three key areas to focus on as we build good health post-menopause:

- Mindset
- Meals
- Movement

These are the 'holy trinity' of the power decade. None of them work alone: there's no point being laser-focused on one but neglecting to develop the others. The good news is we can fit these habits into a busy lifestyle – nothing is difficult or complicated – but it does need focus. Focus on ourselves, our health and what's right for us. This is how the three Ms stack up:

Mindset: If we're unhappy or living in a state of constant stress, we simply can't power up: the healthiest diet and the best exercise regime are nothing without a happy, healthy mind. We need to feel good about ourselves, to prioritise and seek ways to rest and relax. Part of this is being able, and willing, to advocate for ourselves, to take our seat at the table and articulate our needs. It's time to find our sense of purpose, knowing WHY we want to take charge of our health and what the benefits will be long term.

Meals: Getting nutrition right in the power decade may just need a few tweaks, or a radical overhaul of how you eat. Either way, I'll guide you through the best way to eat (and drink) to make the most of this time. Fundamentally, it means a reliance on fresh produce and home-prepared meals, giving ourselves the best, most nutritionally-dense foods without loading up on unnecessary refined carbohydrates and processed foods. It also means enjoying our food, not punishing ourselves with restrictive diets or cutting out a food group. We need to nourish ourselves in a way that's sustainable long term while supporting the best possible health.

Movement: Nothing makes more difference to short- and long-term health outcomes than movement. It doesn't have to be 'exercise' or 'a workout'; just moving our bodies makes a massive difference to how we feel in our power decade. Our bodies are designed to move, but modern life is designed to keep us static, at our desks or on our sofas. Something has to give: we have to find a way of working regular, varied movement into our lives.

These three themes weave throughout the book – look out for simple daily actions you can use to transform your health in each section.

SECTION 3 covers how we can power up our body and mind. This is where we delve into some of the issues you could be experiencing right now, persistent symptoms which may have accompanied you into the post-menopausal years. Every single woman has a very different experience, but there are some constants.

Sleep: We need to get our sleep right – the modern world is designed to keep us awake and we've learned not to prioritise sleep in the way we should. But lack of sleep can have a serious knock-on effect on our health as we age, increasing our risk of dementia and heart disease.

Genitourinary syndrome and menopause: This section of the book has been such an eye-opener for me. The decline in our reproductive hormones can have a lasting impact on our pelvic health, giving rise to vulval, vaginal and urinary symptoms that can stay with us for the rest of our lives, unless we confront them.

Other persistent physical symptoms: Some of the issues we think of as menopausal can stay with us for many years afterwards. We'll look at vasomotor symptoms (hot flushes and night sweats) as well as other longer-term issues like aches and pains, dry eyes, hearing difficulties, dry skin, dry mouth and dental health problems.

Stress: That feeling of being overwhelmed, unable to cope with mental or emotional pressure, can play a huge role in perimenopausal symptoms, and it doesn't disappear post-menopause (unfortunately). Our power decade may be a time of personal growth and joy, but we may also experience some of the most stressful events of our lives in this period. The good news is we can work to change our response to stress, and give ourselves the tools to ride out the events that threaten to overwhelm us.

Persistent mental and emotional symptoms of menopause: I talk to so many women who've found a pervading sense of anxiety has seeped into their fifties and sixties. It may have started in their perimenopausal years, it may be a new addition to a suite of symptoms exacerbated by stress and the complexities of midlife. Low libido, brain fog and difficulties handling change can all be part of the mental and emotional experience of these years.

SECTION 4 puts the controls in your hands, showing you how to reduce the risk of long-term health issues you may not be experiencing right now. There is a very clear path (well, more of a six-lane highway) from the changes of menopause to the chronic diseases of ageing that can kick in ten to fifteen years later. We need to use the time in between the two wisely, because we're not getting it back. I'll show you how small daily habits will help you to:

Manage weight and insulin resistance: It's a rare woman who doesn't experience changes to weight and body shape during the menopause transition and beyond. Declining oestrogen alters how our bodies respond to carbohydrate and causes us to store body fat differently. More seriously, we're more likely to become insulin resistant (a precursor to type 2 diabetes).

Heart your heart: Alzheimer's and dementia may have overtaken heart disease as the biggest killer of women in the UK,[3] but it's still a major risk factor for women. Oestrogen protects the lining of our artery walls by reducing the build-up of plaque. As oestrogen declines through the peri-menopause and beyond, our coronary arteries are more likely to narrow, resulting in stiffer blood vessels and an increased risk of heart attack and stroke.

Boost bone health: Oestrogen regulates bone remodelling and turnover, so as this hormone declines, so does the strength of our bones. Without it, they're more likely to weaken and break. Fractures can have a devastating impact on our health as we age: keeping our bones resilient, and preventing falls, can vastly improve our quality of life.

Build a better brain: Research shows that hormonal changes brought about by menopause physically remodel our brains. Their energy consumption is different post-menopause. We may – or may not – have emerged from perimenopausal brain fog, but during this decade we need to work hard to keep our brains wiring and firing.

Douse inflammation: One of the key drivers of ageing and poor health, inflammation is exacerbated by lower oestrogen levels post-menopause. Add in the fact that we live in an inflamed world: our inflammation levels rise in response to our environment, to processed foods, pollution, toxins and more. But inflammation responds well to a healthy lifestyle and we can lower our levels.

A word about cancer risk: Cancer risk increases with age, regardless of gender or menopausal status. Our risk can be predetermined by genetics, early life or just bad luck, but it's important we know the risks and the lifestyle measures we can take to reduce it. It's particularly important we're aware of our risks of breast and gynaecological cancers.

Finally, look out for interviews scattered throughout the book with women who are thriving in their own power decade. They're all building the life they want in their fifties and beyond, with good health – physical and mental – at the centre of it. They've also found ways to share their experiences and help others as they go. Meet the **Power Women**:

- Fay Reid
- Jacqueline Hooton
- Jo McEwan and Ann Stephens from Positive Pause

- Jo Moseley
- Kanan Thakerar
- Karen Arthur
- Rachel Lankester
- Tracy Acock

There's so much negative messaging about life after menopause: these women reject the narrative that it's the start of a slippery slope into decrepitude and old age. It isn't. They're all creating bright, powerful futures for themselves, using their own experience of the menopause transition as a springboard to a new and thrilling life.

What Just Happened?
The Menopause

Congratulations, you're post-menopausal! Sounds simple, right? But there's a lot to unpack here. Most obviously, we can no longer get pregnant (although don't come off birth control until you've discussed it with your doctor). This is a huge relief to some, a source of profound sadness for others. And, as we reach menopause, we are confronted by our own mortality: our ageing self is waiting for us on the other side. Which is precisely why our power decade – the first ten or so years we are post-menopause – is so vital for our health.

MENOPAUSE: THE FACTS

The menopause itself is just one day. Technically, that's it. It's the day we get our last period, but can only be defined retrospectively, once we haven't had another period for a year. We can't predict the date in advance. And, of course, a lot of women don't know when their last period occurs because they're on contraception, HRT or have had a hysterectomy. In the years leading up to that day, we may experience physiological and psychological symptoms, starting in our late thirties. Those years are defined as perimenopause, and often feel like a rollercoaster of surging and waning hormones.

When perimenopause begins, how long it lasts and how severe the symptoms are is impacted by genetics, health – obesity and smoking, for example – and factors such as race, ethnicity and socioeconomic status.[4] The Study of Women's Health Across the Nation[5] (SWAN) surveyed over 3,000 middle-aged women in the USA and found that 80 per cent experienced vasomotor symptoms – the hot flushes and night sweats so often associated with the menopause transition. The median duration of these symptoms was 7.4 years. That's a lot of hot flushes and night sweats. Duration was strongly influenced by race and ethnicity, with Black women experiencing the longest symptoms (10.1 years) and Japanese-American women the shortest (4.8 years). Black women were also more likely to have a longer transition, starting at a younger age and experiencing more severe symptoms. Health inequalities can mean that ethnically diverse women are also less likely to have access to the support and medical care they may need during the menopause transition.

The average age of menopause in the UK is fifty-one.[6] That means some women experience it in their forties, as I did, while others are still having regular periods in their late fifties. We are, as always, all different. Before the age of forty-five, it's known as early menopause. Before the age of forty, the terms premature menopause or pre-mature ovarian insufficiency (POI) are used. This affects one in a hundred women.[7] Many women will have a surgical menopause, which follows immediately after a bi-lateral oophorectomy (removal of both ovaries). This abrupt menopause is likely to cause more severe symptoms than when hormones decline naturally. If the ovaries remain intact following a hysterectomy, menopause is likely to occur within about five years.[8] Around one in five women in the UK will have a hysterectomy during their lives.

34+ MENOPAUSE SYMPTOMS

I'm thrilled beyond belief about the 'Menopause Revolution': the powerful movement focused on giving women the help and support they need from the start of perimenopause. This phase of our lives comes with often debilitating symptoms and for too long has been – and remains – under-discussed and under-treated for so many. I applaud and salute the doctors and individual women who've taken a stand and kickstarted that revolution.

This book is not about perimenopause: it's about the years after we reach that 'one day' and how we create good health POST-menopause. But we can only do that if we understand what happened to our bodies, and our health, during the peri years. And many, many of us will take perimenopausal symptoms into the 'post-' years. Oh, the joy.

If you're coming to this book post-menopause, you'll likely know your own symptoms. But the menopause transition affects women in so many different ways that the first time I saw a list of possible symptoms I found myself thinking, 'Ahhhh, so that's menopause, huh?' There are many symptoms listed below that I thought were just 'life after forty', but which turned out to be directly caused by the hormonal changes I was experiencing. My symptoms were manageable, but some women are driven by theirs to leave jobs and relationships, or even to suicide: our own symptoms, and those of others, should never be taken lightly.

It used to be that doctors thought there were three major symptoms of menopause: irregular periods, hot flushes and night sweats. Now it's recognised that there are at least thirty-four, and even this list isn't exhaustive. I've seen lists with fifty-four symptoms, but in the interests of brevity I'm sharing thirty-four here. Every woman has a different transition, and wildly varying symptoms. But they're all a direct result of the dramatic changes our bodies go through as levels of reproductive hormones – oestrogen, progesterone and testosterone – decline. And this process can have a hugely debilitating impact on our quality of life.

According to the British Menopause Society, more than 75 per cent of women experience symptoms, with 'a quarter describing their symptoms as severe. A third experience long-term symptoms, which may last as much as seven years or longer.'[9]

These are some of the most common symptoms:

1. Irregular periods
2. Hot flushes – the 'classic' symptom, defined medically as a 'vasomotor' symptom
3. Night sweats – another vasomotor symptom
4. Mood swings
5. Anxiety
6. Fatigue
7. Depression
8. Disturbed sleep
9. Decreased libido
10. Irritability
11. Joint pain
12. Brain fog
13. Difficulty concentrating
14. Weight gain
15. Breast tenderness
16. Headaches
17. Vaginal dryness
18. Pins and needles or tingling, particularly in hands and feet
19. Dry or burning mouth
20. Changes in taste
21. Bloating
22. Digestive issues
23. Muscle aches
24. Electric shock sensations

25. Itchiness
26. Thinning hair
27. Brittle nails
28. Stress incontinence
29. Dizziness
30. Allergies
31. Osteoporosis
32. Irregular heartbeat, or palpitations
33. Increased body odour
34. Panic attacks

There's a really good symptom tracker on the Menopause Support website if you need more help on this – see menopausesupport.co.uk.

WHAT CAUSES THESE SYMPTOMS?

Women are born with a finite number of eggs, all metaphorically lined up and waiting in our ovaries. Following the hormonal maelstrom that is puberty, the ovaries release one egg each month (usually) to either make a baby or to pass through our uterus unfertilised – until the supply starts to run out. And that's when the fun starts.

The oestrogen needed to power puberty, and then a monthly cycle for several decades, is controlled by the hypothalamus.[10] This tiny structure, deep in the brain, regulates emotions, temperature, appetite, circadian rhythms, growth, stress, sleep and, most importantly for us here, hormones. The hypothalamus is connected to the pituitary gland, which secretes reproductive hormones into our bloodstream. Two of these are particularly important: the follicle-stimulating hormone (FSH) and luteinising hormone (LH). They work in harmony, controlling our menstrual cycle by telling the ovaries to release an egg each month and to create oestrogen and progesterone, the main reproductive hormones. As egg supplies run low, the hypothalamus and pituitary gland ramp up production of FSH and LH to try to crank up the ovaries, causing hormones to go haywire.

What makes this all the more difficult is that the hypothalamus has a co-dependent relationship with oestrogen. The hypothalamus both controls the hormones that lead to oestrogen production and responds to oestrogen itself.[11] When oestrogen supplies run low the hypothalamus' temperature control short-circuits. Hence the hot flushes and night sweats that so many women experience during the menopause transition. And that's not all our plummeting oestrogen levels have in store for us.

WHAT HAS OESTROGEN EVER DONE FOR US?

We have to understand that oestrogen is not just a hormone of reproduction: we have receptors for it throughout our bodies. It affects the urinary tract, heart and blood vessels, bones, breasts, skin, hair, mucous membranes, pelvic muscles and – critically – the brain. This is an extremely reductive way of looking at it, but during our reproductive years, oestrogen wraps us in a protective cloak: it keeps us healthy so we're able to make species-perpetuating babies. Which makes total sense from an evolutionary standpoint.

During our reproductive years, our bodies run on a type of oestrogen called estradiol. Having too much of it can result in acne, loss of sex drive, osteoporosis and depression. Too little leaves us at risk of weight gain and cardiovascular disease. But when levels are just right it keeps us in good reproductive, bone, brain and cardiovascular health.

Estradiol is an all-round good guy (girl?) in our pre-menopausal bodies. This self-made wonder-drug supports bone growth, promoting the activity of osteoblasts, the cells that make new bone. It protects the heart, particularly the inner layer of the artery wall, where it helps keep blood vessels flexible. It also reduces our risk of obesity by regulating metabolism and fat stores. The lubrication of our joints comes from estradiol, keeping them comfortable and moving. It also affects the production of collagen, which plays a role in maintaining joint cartilage and skin tone.

In addition, estradiol has a vital effect on both our cognitive and mental health. Cerebral blood flow and neuronal activity are increased by oestrogen, protecting our brain and stimulating the production of new neurons. It also acts on the parts of the brain that control emotion, stimulating the production of serotonin and endorphins, both 'feelgood' chemicals.

It also has a profound effect on how we perceive ourselves. Oestrogen helps us nurture, putting the needs of others before our own. In her interview on page 265, Rachel Lankester describes it as 'the biddable hormone', the one that keeps us looking out for others. When oestrogen levels decline, we're more minded to put ourselves first and meet our own needs: a key component of the power decade.

Post-menopause, we still make oestrogen, but in a weaker form known as estrone. It's created in the adrenal glands and in body fat. It's able to force the body to store fat in new places, such as the stomach area. And estrone lacks estradiol's power to protect our brains, bones and hearts. Which is precisely why we need to step up and take control of our own health in the decade post-menopause.

OTHER HORMONES IMPACTED BY MENOPAUSE

Of course, oestrogen doesn't act alone. It works in harmony with the other reproductive hormones – progesterone and testosterone, both of which are made in the ovaries during our fertile years.

Progesterone is the dominant hormone in the second phase of our menstrual cycle, helping manage the uterus lining by preparing it for a fertilised egg or sweeping it away if there isn't one. More importantly at this phase in our lives, it's known as a 'calming hormone' because it enhances mood and reduces the risk of depression. It's also linked to sleep quality and lower levels of anxiety.

Testosterone isn't just a male hormone (although men have ten times as much as women). Produced in the ovaries and adrenals, it helps regulate sex drive, energy levels and fat distribution. All things that can go awry during perimenopause and beyond. Testosterone is linked to better mood, more energy and sharper brain function, as well as raising levels of the feel good hormone dopamine in the brain. It also increases libido and improves orgasm.

Like oestrogen, progesterone and testosterone stimulate bone formation and slow bone loss. And all three of the reproductive hormones impact other hormones: cortisol, the stress hormone; insulin, which manages blood sugar levels; and both serotonin and dopamine, which regulate mood. They are all in constant contact with the hypothalamus and pituitary gland in the brain, working in harmony to keep our bodies and minds on an even keel. Until . . . they don't, and that's when the symptoms of perimenopause kick in.

THE GRANDMOTHER HYPOTHESIS

Yes, reproductive hormones are very powerful, but we're designed to live without them. We're unusual among species on this planet because human females just keep going when our reproductive days are over. Females of other species tend to shuffle off when baby-making ends.

We don't. This is the basis of the 'grandmother hypothesis': an anthropological concept that explains the survival of post-reproductive women. Grandmothers, it's hypothesised, are needed to care for the young and thus perpetuate their genes. In traditional societies, like the Hadza in Tanzania, grandmothers are also the most adept foragers, gathering more food for the tribe than they consume themselves.[12]

But what if you're still suffering menopause symptoms when you're well into your peak foraging years?

I'M NOT HAVING PERIODS, BUT I'M STILL HAVING SYMPTOMS

I don't know about you, but I don't miss periods one bit. I look at my daughters (aged twenty-one and nineteen as I write this) and feel nothing but sympathy for the cramps, hot-water-bottle-hugging and tampon hoarding required to get through a monthly cycle. That takes a huge amount of energy – energy that has now been freed up for our power decade. It's very liberating.

But just because we're no longer having periods doesn't mean we're not having menopause symptoms. The SWAN study mentioned on page 18 found that, of the median 7.4 years that vasomotor (hot flushes, night sweats etc.) symptoms persisted, 4.5 of those years were after the final menstrual period (FMP). That's a long time after the hot-water-bottle-hugging years to be experiencing menopause symptoms.

27

Research in Australia found that more than 15 per cent of post-menopausal women aged fifty-five to fifty-nine were still suffering moderate to severe vasomotor symptoms, as were 6.5 per cent of post-menopausal women aged sixty to sixty-five.[13] Smokers and women who were overweight were more likely to still be suffering.

Severe symptoms post-menopause have also been linked to high levels of anxiety. A study of 3,500 Latin American women found that post-menopausal women with anxiety were five times more likely to suffer severe physical symptoms post-menopause than those without anxiety.[14]

You might be wondering if menopause symptoms ever end. For the majority of women they do, tailing off in the years after that FMP. But we should not underestimate the long-term impact of the decline in hormones on our health post-menopause. Hot flushes, for example, may wane, but our bone, brain and heart health are at risk if we don't look after ourselves (there's more on this in Section 4).

If you are suffering from the symptoms listed above – or any other unexplained symptoms that are having a detrimental impact on your day-to-day life – please talk to your doctor. It doesn't matter if your final menstrual period was years ago, or if you haven't reached it yet – you deserve to get the help and support you need. Ask your GP about whether hormone replacement therapy (HRT), also known as menopause therapy (MT), is right for you. Ask about lifestyle interventions that will help relieve your symptoms and look at the list of resources at the end of this book. Some women suffer for years before they get the right help. There is still a huge amount to be done to spread the word that, for many women, menopause symptoms can be relieved quickly and safely.

To quote the medical journal *The Lancet*:

> *For too long, women's healthcare needs at menopause have been under-recognised and underserved by the healthcare profession [. . .] education, support and access to treatments for menopausal symptom relief and prevention of later-life chronic diseases must be available to all women irrespective of race, ethnicity, socioeconomic status or geographical location. With such a foundation in place, women will be able to go through the menopause with confidence, embrace the next chapter of their lives and lead longer and healthier lives.*

Yes! This book is all about embracing that next chapter and ensuring we use it as a springboard for that longer, healthier life.

DO I NEED HRT?

I'm not a doctor, so I can't advise on, or prescribe, a medication like HRT. As a health coach and writer, I can share what I know: my own experience, that of my clients and what I learned from the wonderful menopause-specialist doctors

I interviewed for this book. Most of all, I would urge you to do your own research, talk to your own doctor – and if you're not happy with their response, ask for a referral. Dr Carys Sonnenberg advises, 'It is so important to educate yourself about all the options available to help manage your symptoms. With knowledge gained from trusted sources, you can make a balanced, informed decision on what is best for you. We are all individual; if you feel your hormones are changing then they probably are, you know your body best.'

Hormone replacement therapy is the single best medical intervention if you are suffering menopause symptoms. That doesn't mean you have to take it, or want to take it, or that it will be right for you. You may be strongly advised not to take it, if you have a history of breast cancer, or certain other medical issues. If you have early menopause, or primary ovarian insufficiency (POI), you will most likely be strongly advised to take it to support your health, at least until the average age of menopause.

What is clear is that for too long both women and doctors were in the dark about the benefits of HRT to relieve the symptoms of menopause. Too many women have either not sought help, or have been sent away from their doctors with 'you're too young/old to be in menopause' ringing in their ears. Or 'but you're still having periods, you can't be menopausal' or 'HRT is dangerous' or many other things.

In autumn 2022, the British Menopause Society published the following information for doctors:

> *The decision whether to take HRT, the dose and duration of its use should be made on an individualised basis after discussing the benefits and risks with each patient. This should be considered in the context of the overall benefits obtained from using HRT including symptom control and improving quality of life as well as considering the bone and cardiovascular benefits associated with HRT use. Discussions with women should also cover aspects such as when to consider stopping HRT and how this can be done (by gradually reducing the dose of HRT). No arbitrary limits should be set on age or duration of HRT intake.*

HRT should be considered as part of a healthy lifestyle: it's not an either/or situation. Dr Juliet Balfour told me, 'There's this idea that you can have HRT and just carry on having a terrible lifestyle. But it's so important to talk about lifestyle as well. This is a really good time to look at what you can do to improve your long-term health.'

HAVE I MISSED THE BOAT?

A client confided she was worried she 'had missed the boat' on HRT because she wasn't offered it at the time of her menopause transition, twelve years ago. Now she feels she's surrounded by messaging that HRT is the only way to prevent the chronic conditions of ageing like dementia, osteoporosis and heart disease. But that's not the case – HRT can have benefits, but the most important thing we can do at this stage of life is look after ourselves. My client and I agreed we would find her a new boat – one where lifestyle interventions keep her health afloat.

It appears there is a 'window of opportunity' for starting HRT to gain the most health benefits. Dr Juliet Balfour explains: 'The NICE guidelines say that if you start HRT within ten years of your last period or under the age of sixty, the benefits outweigh the risks for most women. This is because the cardiovascular benefits are so great. So if someone wants to start HRT, it's best if we can get them started within ten years of their last period, but ideally a lot sooner than that. Women past this stage can certainly still consider HRT for symptom control, looking at their individual benefits versus risks with their doctor. The bone health benefits are seen whatever age HRT is started.'

A lot depends on the severity of menopausal symptoms, regardless of age. There's evidence that HRT also helps with some of the health issues of the post-menopausal years, such as heart disease risk and bone density depletion. But it's not for everyone, and it's not a 'magic pill' that will make the health issues of our fifties, sixties and beyond disappear. HRT may give us back hormones, but it doesn't give us back the resilience of youth. There's also a small risk of breast cancer with long-term (over five years) use with some types of HRT,[15] which you should discuss with your doctor.

Also be aware that guidelines on the use of HRT are updated regularly as new research is published. It's a rapidly changing field: stay informed, keep reading and talk to your doctor if you want more guidance.

'Watch this space,' says Dr Balfour, 'things are changing all the time as we get new evidence.'

Three Actions to Kickstart Your Power Decade

The menopause transition for many women is a daunting time of change, of unexpected health challenges, of roller-coaster emotions and unprecedented shifts in how we feel physically and emotionally. But we emerge wiser than before, and stronger than we know. This is the time to step away from the prevailing narrative of failing faculties and oncoming illness and instead power up to make the changes that will define how we age. From now, for the rest of our lives . . .

Start the process of creating your own power decade by committing to these three actions:

UNDERSTAND THE SCIENCE AND HOW IT CAN HELP YOU

This has been a game changer for me in terms of motivation to keep looking after myself. It's one thing to think, 'I need to exercise to keep fit'; it's another thing to know, 'I need to exercise because new research shows that strength training helps post-menopausal women manage hot flushes, reduce their dementia risk and stabilise glucose'. And, similarly, we know we need to eat vegetables but it's much more inspiring – and we're much more likely to do it – when we know how they keep our bodies and brains healthy. It's on us to use the knowledge that's freely available to make the best of our own health, to stay informed and up to date.

TRACK YOUR STATS

As above, knowledge is power. The more we know about what's going on in our bodies, the more we can modify what needs to change. If you have a test at the doctor's (and see below for what you could ask for), keep a record of the results. If you weigh yourself, or measure your body mass index (BMI), keep a note. There's an NHS BMI tracker app that explains the equation needed to calculate body mass index and helps monitor changes over time. I keep a folder on my computer where I can save any information I get from the doctor, like blood pressure and cholesterol levels. If we take ownership of our health, are proactive and know our numbers, we're more likely to thrive and to stay motivated to make changes.

There's also a huge range of apps and wearable devices available to help us keep track of our health. I love my Oura ring, others are big Fitbit fans, and any smart phone will give you the basics of how much you're moving each day. Harness the technology and make it work for you.

GET TESTED

It's up to us to take responsibility for our health, and remember doctors are there to support us in that. If you're offered a test by the doctor, take it! The NHS health check is offered to people over forty in most parts of the UK and covers the main tests we need. It's designed to spot early risk for stroke, kidney disease, heart disease, type-2 diabetes and dementia. Tests offered vary across the UK (and across the world), but we should have regular tests for:

- Blood pressure – aim for blood pressure between 90/60 and 120/80
- Cholesterol levels – total cholesterol should be below 5
- Blood sugar – your blood sugar level should be below 42
- BMI – aim for between 18.5 and 24.9
- Mammogram and cervical smear tests
- Bowel cancer screening – if you're over sixty you should be offered a faecal immunochemical test

At time of writing, the UK All-Party Parliament Group (APPG) on Menopause has called for a free NHS health check at forty-five for all women to discuss menopause and HRT. MP Carolyn Harris, chair of the APPG, said, 'We are beginning to feel the tide of change but the taboo around the menopause still prevails in all corners of society – in workplaces, within families and among friends, in education, and in the medical profession.' Hopefully, these health checks will be put in place soon. If you need help with menopausal symptoms your doctor should be your first port of call.

How Do You Feel Right Now?

I want this book to make you feel as if you've got a health coach in your pocket, or your bag, or on your bedside table. Remember that I'm with you, rooting for you and willing you on.

One of the most powerful tools in coaching is to track progress. You can't improve what you don't track. Keep a record of where you are now, where you want to go and how you're going to get there. Let's end this section with a check-in.

- What are your health concerns right now?
- Are you experiencing menopausal symptoms? Hot flushes, night sweats, brain fog, genitourinary symptoms etc.? (see list on p. 21)
- What are your long-term health concerns? Heart disease, dementia, arthritis, cancer?
- What is a typical day's food and drink for you? List meals, snacks and drinks.
- How often do you exercise per week, and what form of exercise do you take?

- How many hours' sleep do you get on average?
- Do you feel stress in your life? If so, why?
- Do you do anything to mitigate against stress?
- Do you feel you have a sense of purpose? What gets you up in the morning?
- Do you feel that you're thriving? If not, what would it take to get you there?

When I asked some of these questions of the thousands of followers of The Age-Well Project, the answers were as varied as the women who wrote them.

My (highly unscientific) survey showed there is no 'normal' in our fifties and sixties – around one third of respondents weren't suffering menopause-related symptoms, either because they were on HRT, had simply left their symptoms behind, or had experienced very few as they went through the transition. Others were still experiencing symptoms, with insomnia, night sweats and brain fog forming an 'unholy trinity' of the most common.

Some felt weighed down by the process of ageing, and the health concerns that come with it. Some felt the decades post-menopause were a time of freedom. Here are a couple of my favourite responses:

'This stage of life is a time to enjoy. It's a time to seize opportunities and try new experiences.'

And: 'I'm more confident, don't have to answer to anyone, feel free to do what I want, no periods which is a bonus. I am enjoying this stage of my life.'

I hope this can be you too.

Power Women: Fay Reid

Fay, 55, set up the brilliant, and much-needed, 9 to 5 Menopause project to share her experience as a Black woman and to offer working women of all ethnicities education, tips and resources. She collaborates with businesses and NHS departments to develop menopause policies and training. She made this midlife career pivot after her own, difficult, menopause transition where she felt unable to ask for support at work.

Fay's symptoms came as a complete shock. She was in the first week of a new job as PA to the CEO of a hugely successful business when she had her first hot flush. 'My menopause initially was one of complete ignorance. When it happened a few more times I thought, "oh, that must be a hot flush" and I laughed to myself because I thought – at forty-five – I was very young. My perception of menopause was old White ladies wearing beige clothing. I said nothing to management about what I was experiencing. I was scared of how people would perceive me, scared they'd think I was really old.'

Fay's symptoms worsened when the business she worked for was about to be sold, and her mother was diagnosed with terminal cancer. 'Those two things were big triggers. My symptoms imploded and I slowly started to fall apart. I had insomnia, I had severe anxiety. Getting up five days a week when you've not slept the night before and doing an hour and a half commute and getting into work, trying to feel switched on enough to support the CEO, was challenging. I never talked about it to anyone at work. I started seeing a therapist because I was spiralling, thinking I was losing the plot. She suggested I see my GP about my symptoms and I was lucky – they gave me HRT straight off the bat. We tried several different types before I had the eureka moment and realised that I felt different, I felt better. And from that point on I was able to deal with things a bit more.'

Fay started to do more research, looking for support. 'I found nobody who had a job and nobody who looked like me talking about menopause. The women who were talking about menopause were affluent, White and they didn't have jobs. They recommended personal nutritionists and private clinics. I thought, "I can't be the only one with a job going through this. I can't be the only Black woman going through this." That was my thought process. And my Instagram account @9to5menopause started from that point. When I was going through perimenopause I was going out, I was dating, I was buying clothes – I wanted to look good and make an effort with my skincare, make-up and hair. My Instagram account started because I wanted to share what I was doing to help myself, and because I have a job, I'm Black and I'm not old.'

The account took off and Fay started gathering followers. 'One thing I noticed is that with the Caribbean and African communities they don't talk about menopause, although that is starting to change. I noticed that Black women would follow me but wouldn't necessarily interact with me, whereas White women were more forthcoming. But it's slowly changing. One thing I found is Black women are more likely to struggle on and not say anything. Looking back, I could tell when my mum was going through menopause, but she never mentioned the word.'

I asked Fay what she says to women in the workplace who are in menopause. 'I encourage them to talk about it – talk to trusted colleagues at work, talk to your friends, to your family. Don't hide it under the carpet, don't be scared. Get information; that made such a difference to me. I'm the living embodiment of feeling good and functioning.'

Fay's new career as a workplace menopause trainer grew out of the success of 9 to 5 Menopause. 'Primarily it was just a hobby for me to share my tips, but as it went along people asked me to speak at events, to appear on podcasts. And when the business I worked for sold, I decided to concentrate on 9 to 5 Menopause. When women step forward and thank me, and tell me that they've found my talks very informative, it gives me a fuzzy glow. And even if I can make one woman feel better, that's good, isn't it? I get to make a difference, and that has pushed me along to make a change in my life.'

When Fay talks to businesses she's clear on how their menopause policy needs to work. 'I push for companies to weave it into their DNA. Let's make it commonplace; we don't have to whisper about menopause. I also advocate for men to be aware of menopause, because we forget that a man might have a partner at home who's really suffering, so his sleep is unsettled too. He could be going to work stressed, not knowing what's going on with his partner. His work performance could also suffer. That's why the awareness needs to be across the board and not just targeted at women. And we can't forget medical menopause, hysterectomy, cancer, endometriosis, trans people in menopause. All these issues should inform our response. And it could be someone in their twenties, not necessarily their forties or fifties.'

Fay continues: 'I'm massively stepping outside my comfort zone doing this. Last week I was on a live panel with a prominent MP and the chief executive of the FTSE Women Leaders Review. When I do events like that I think of my mum, and how proud she would be. Last year, on World Menopause Day, I was on *ITV News* live. Things like that have given me a sense of achievement. Five years ago, it wouldn't have been an option – I was just paddling along, doing a nine-to-five job. I've been given opportunities which have completely petrified me, but I've taken them. They give me a sense of achievement. I feel like I'm entering a new chapter and celebrating the next stage of me.'

Find Fay at www.fayreid.com and @9to5menopause on Instagram.

Power Women: Jacqueline Hooton

Jacqueline, 59, is a personal trainer who runs fitness classes for women in a gym built in her own back garden. Her Instagram account, @hergardengym, has a massive following thanks to her brilliant posts, which skewer ageist narratives and give fantastic health and fitness advice for women in midlife and beyond. Her reels on disrupting ageism have accumulated over 40 million views and seen her featured in the national press.

I asked Jacqueline what had motivated her to get involved with the conversation on ageism. 'Probably, like many women, my first experiences around ageism were as I hit my forties,' she replies. 'I was suddenly aware of some of the attitudes and comments I was getting. I'd always worked in fitness, so I didn't think there would be an expectation that I should change the clothes I was wearing and the activities I was doing and my attitudes in general, just because I'd reached a certain age.

'I've become more incensed with ageism as I've got older. It starts off with a small trickle and gets louder and louder. And although I joke about elements of it, I'm really concerned about the health implications. When women have poor expectations around age and midlife, when they don't feel as valued, there's no balance to the conversation. I don't mean to be controversial, but if we internalise the idea that our forties onwards is a time of decline, we're not going to put the work in to look after ourselves. It's about challenging and changing that narrative because we know it isn't true. We're bombarded with negative images and a negative narrative around ageing: if you search for stock images of women over sixty, it's going to bring up images of women in nursing homes, women with a walking stick, women who look more like my grandmother did. Without even realising it, you've been exposed to this bias, this idea of age for so long, that you might not even be aware of the alternatives, or the actions that can make a difference to your future health trajectory.'

Jacqueline urges us to work to improve our fitness and wellbeing, even if we face health challenges. 'If we can't solve the health issue we're dealing with, we can still be the best version of that. So even if we're dealing with a serious diagnosis, fitness will always support the healthiest version of that. I had an osteoarthritis diagnosis at the beginning of the year so I'm having to adapt too. Fitness isn't just for the super-fit; we can all benefit. I think many women in midlife have watched older parents deteriorate and that's been a bit of a wake-up call. They're worried about their future too; they want to be able to travel, they want to have a healthy retirement. Drill down into what's important then look at what's achievable. Could you go for a ten-minute walk today? What's the low-hanging fruit?'

Growing her Instagram account, particularly in the last two years, has brought with it a sense of responsibility. 'I know there's a lot of confusion and I try to bring balance with what I say. But with more followers, you're going to get people with very different views. And with the issue of ageism and ageist narratives you're challenging their bias, what they think of the world and how women should be. I've always had a lot of different media attention for one reason or another. When I was fifty, I was a mum of five competing in bodybuilding competitions. Now I've had several reels go viral – one I made in summer 2022 has had over 10 million views. I was making fun of the comments people say to you online as a 59-year-old woman, like "You'd look better if you dyed your grey hair" and "You must embarrass your children". I think my reels cause a bit of a Marmite effect, with people either thinking, "Here's a woman saying what I need to hear", or "What on earth? This is terrible." But it pays to be distinctive. Although someone might try to smack you down, there's still a whole raft of women out there who want to stay fit and active.

'I definitely feel positive about approaching sixty, and the future, but that's tempered with a bit of realism as well because I'm going to have to make some adaptations myself. I've got osteoarthritis, I've got a problem with neuroma in my feet, I've had three shoulder surgeries, so there's always something else to work around. I think that attitude is important because my audience is dealing with a lot of different health issues too.

'So much of this is about that sense of responsibility for our own health. Rather than going to the doctor and saying, "Fix me", we need to think how we can fix ourselves and how we can support ourselves. I'm aiming to get to 100 in good health and independent, not being a burden on my children, not being a burden on society, and living my life.'

Find Jacqueline at www.hergardengym.co.uk and @hergardengym on Instagram and Facebook.

SECTION 2

HOW TO HAVE A POWER DECADE

Introduction

This is when we start to thrive. It's time to embrace the adventure of the power decade, making the most of our post-menopausal years. No adventure is too big or too small; just make it yours. It's a privilege to have got this far, so let's own it.

The post-menopause years can be a time of seismic shifts – empty nests, re-evaluated careers, losses and gains as individual as we are. The decade that takes us from our mid-fifties to mid-sixties is a time for us to take stock, to forge ahead, to decide who we are and how we want to live as we face the future. And all this rests on a foundation of the best-possible health.

This is where my 'three Ms' – mindset, meals and movement – come in. They're the holy trinity of post-menopausal health, working together to help you power up in your fifties and beyond.

There's a dedicated chapter for each of the 'three Ms' in this section. I've woven in interviews with experts to guide you through, and added coaching questions from my own 'toolbox' to get you thinking about how you can take action in your own life.

Mindset

Our power decade is about creating the life we want, with good health at its heart. And that has to mean mental health as well as physical. Oestrogen is a comfort blanket that supports positivity and happiness: when it's gone we need to create our own replacement. But we can do it!

Our fifties and sixties may not come with an unending supply of post-menopausal zest: they are times of profound change, bringing with them any possible combination of issues. Or all of them. During these years, my clients often tell me they feel that they've lost themselves, or that they are at the bottom of a long list of other priorities. Many put caring for the wellbeing of others before their own. But this is the time to seek positives and to embrace change. Menopause is a transformation that gifts us the art of self-reflection and the strength to know who we are. That's why putting yourself first is the number one action in this section.

The mindset change that has really made a difference to how I take care of myself, and power up for the years ahead, is drilling down into my own 'purpose'. I've spent a lot of time working out what I want my future to look and feel like. For me, it's about ageing well, reducing my dementia risk and having the faculties to enjoy time with my family and friends. What is it for you? Have a look at point two below to help you find your own purpose.

My guide through this section is menopause expert and coach Meera Bhogal, whose own experience of menopause, which included managing brutal symptoms, has led her to help many hundreds of women through the transition. She found her way through her symptoms, and maintained her health post-menopause, by hunting for answers. 'I don't like having problems; I like having solutions. I didn't like feeling like that. It wasn't me. It wasn't the person that I am. That was the ignition that got me started, but actually what keeps you going is the fact that things start to work, and you see the consistency with which it works.'

Having a positive mindset is a vital part of this: 'It's an internal way of setting your compass at being happy and fulfilled. It takes time and practice. Consistency. Also you need to move away from believing that life is all "happy and rosy". Apply equanimity to good and bad situations and realise that it's all part of our journey.'

Meera finds particular issues around menopause and mindset within her own South Asian community: 'Because of the culture, because of the way women's health is just not talked about, I quite often speak to women who would like to do more to support their health through menopause but who can't because of their families. There's this expectation of them as women not to be selfish, because taking care of your health can be seen as selfish; you're expected to put up with it and get on with it. So there are a lot of taboos we have to break, lots of myths we have to bust before women can get to the point where they don't get resistance from their families, and their own communities.'

Find Meera at meerabhogal.com and @meerabhogal on Instagram.

TEN WAYS TO POWER UP YOUR MINDSET

1. Put Yourself First

If you're flicking through this book thinking, 'This is all very well, Susan, but I don't have time to exercise/cook from scratch/prioritise sleep', take a step back for a moment. What are you making time for? I know it's going to be something very valid – a demanding job or caring responsibilities, for example. But the actions in this book will help make you better at the thing that is taking your time. If you start to see a healthy lifestyle as an extension of the other priorities in your life, the perspective changes. As Meera says, 'Sometimes we need to make difficult decisions, because we could be here for another thirty or forty years. You either need to make this a priority or you keep going in this cycle of crash and burn and not actually getting any further forward with your own health. Being "selfish" now is going to help you be able to give to others more over the years.'

POWER COACHING QUESTION: Ask yourself the difficult question of what happens if your health fails? Who would support the other priorities you have?

2. Purpose

What does your power decade look and feel like? Visualise that wonderful, healthy life you want for yourself. Really see it in your mind's eye, and trust that you will be able to manifest it. Your purpose is to create that life, to manifest it. For Meera, it's simple: 'I don't want to be ill. I want to be around for as long as I can, as healthy as I can. I want to get up in the morning and feel right.' The next step on from that is to align our behaviours so that our life in the present leads us towards the life we want. And the route to that, says Meera, is 'to really get to know yourself. Turn around and reflect on who you are and what type of personality you are. That way you'll understand the kind of help and support you need.'

POWER COACHING QUESTION: What's your purpose? What does your future look like? Start from that point and work backwards to what you need to start doing now.

3. Self-Efficacy

Self-efficacy refers to how we view challenges – either as something to master or a threat to avoid. Having a strong sense of self-efficacy, believing we can rise to those challenges, makes us more likely to be able to manage them, and at lower risk of depression and stress. It's not the same as confidence, it's about having a strong belief that we have the capacity to achieve our goals. Can you see a challenge as an opportunity to grow? We all have a great deal of life experience by now, so we need to reflect on the skills we've learned and the tools we have at our disposal. One of my clients was dealing with a difficult family member. I'd noticed that she's a fantastic prepper – always preparing meals in advance and leaving her desk neat and tidy ready for the next day's work. We applied those skills to the issues she was facing so she prepared for them in advance.

POWER COACHING QUESTION: What's in your toolbox? Ask yourself what strengths you have to count on when facing a difficult situation.

4. Find the Joy

It's easy to get to midlife with a pervading sense that we're so weighed down by responsibility that much of the joy has been sucked out of life. Add to that the hormonal changes of perimenopause and things aren't much fun. But as we leave the transition behind, this is the time to rediscover the joy of life. Remember how much fun we had as kids? Puberty put a lid on that, chaining us to a complex monthly cycle that dictated our moods and actions. Now we can rediscover that sense of freedom. For Meera it's about acknowledging the things you are doing, and who you are now. 'Understand that you're turning into a whole new person as you go through the transition, with a whole new energy and a whole set of different opportunities,' she says. She's seen it with her clients too: 'The number of women I've spoken to who've suddenly found new careers, or new creativity, or they study or do different things, it's absolutely incredible. The joy comes from that freedom.'

POWER COACHING QUESTION: Who is the post-menopausal you? What would bring that person joy?

5. Self-Compassion

By our fifties and sixties we may well have spent a great deal of time caring for others – raising children, mentoring young colleagues, looking after parents or older family members. We learn to show them compassion – but how much do we show ourselves? We tend to be our own harshest critic, punishing ourselves for our mistakes and undervaluing our accomplishments. Meera's clear on the importance of this: 'Being kind to yourself is where it all starts. Put yourself first and you will find things will fall into place; avoid that self-deprecating rhetoric because that in itself is your ego giving importance to the negativity. So let it go by, observe it and allow it to pass without reacting. It gets easier with time and practice.' Be mindful of the difficult emotions that arise and accept that you're not perfect. You're learning and growing all the time, from each experience, and that's a positive thing.

POWER COACHING QUESTION: Can you be your own best mate? If a friend was going through a similar situation, how would you talk to them?

6. Talk to Those Around You

Psychotherapists talk about the importance of giving ourselves a seat at the table. Are you able to say no to some of the demands put upon you? Meera describes saying no as 'one of the biggest things you can do'. Advocating for ourselves and our own needs in a stressful situation is a very powerful response that helps put us back in control. It's about giving ourselves 'agency' – taking action with a particular goal in mind. To do this, it's essential we communicate openly and honestly with those around us. Explaining to others how we feel and the changes we are going through can be enlightening for them and unburdening for us. We talk about menopause as a transition, and transformation, because we experience so much, mentally and physically, during these years. Make sure those around you know where you're at and how you're feeling.

POWER COACHING QUESTION: What would you like the people around you to know about how you feel right now?

7. Who Cares What People Think?

Oestrogen seems to have a way of keeping us in line, so we do what we're supposed to be doing. We worry about what people think of us and our place in the world. When it declines, our perspective shifts. Meera concurs: 'That freedom, the freedom that comes when you just don't care if somebody likes you or doesn't like you, has a lot of joy in it. I only wish we could have had that energy when we were younger; we wouldn't have been bothered by half the things that got us down and made us feel bad.'

POWER COACHING QUESTION: Imagine you're free from all constraints imposed by the opinion of others. What do you do now?

8. Mindfulness: Bring Awareness to Our Thoughts and Choices

The term mindfulness refers to the non-judgemental observations of our thoughts, feelings and actions, which we witness without trying to suppress them. It's often linked to meditation, but it's not the same practice. There's a wonderful Rumi poem called 'The Guest House', which describes our thoughts and feelings as guests that arrive each day.

The poem urges us to welcome each one and see them as a guide to the next stage of our lives. As we go through our day, we welcome many thoughts and make many choices. Seeing our thoughts as separate from us, rather than defining us, is extremely powerful.

POWER COACHING QUESTION: Can you create some objectivity and consider whether your thoughts are helping or hindering you?

9. Get Outside, and Reflect

Let Mother Nature do some of the work. The simple act of going outside gives our brains some much-needed downtime, allowing us a few moments to relax, so we're less likely to keep ruminating on difficult situations. Use the time to ask yourself some reflective questions. Self-reflection is about stepping back from negative thought patterns and trying to work out WHY we feel the way we do, or using that mental space to problem-solve. It can also be about looking at what is working well in our lives. Combine it with a walk outside in the morning to get daylight, which kickstarts our circadian rhythms, and we're winning at life!

POWER COACHING QUESTION: Ask yourself some questions – why do I feel X about Y? What is this telling me? Using questions helps us get a little bit of distance from our thoughts, and allows us to evaluate them better.

10. Get Inspired by Others

The best motivator of all is having someone in your life who shares your goals and outlook. That could be a partner, a friend or a community. Talk to the women around you: who else in your life wants a power decade? Who else is striving to thrive in their fifties and sixties? We all rise together, so the more people you can bring with you on the journey, the better. And if there's someone cheerleading for you on the sidelines, affirming the work that you're putting in and the progress you're making, that's a huge support too. Seek inspiration from women in the media and on socials too – there are so many supportive communities out there. Meera says, 'Women need support. Start searching for a community of people that will be able to support you with factual, non-judgemental information. Then, it's almost like stepping stones. You do that step and then from that step, you'll take another step and another step as you get educated and inspired.'

POWER COACHING QUESTION: Have you read the Power Women interviews woven throughout this book for more inspiration? Learn about women who have lifted me up and how they have created their own power decades.

PUTTING IT ALL TOGETHER

It goes without saying that if your mental health is suffering, please seek professional help. But many of my clients come to me for health coaching in their fifties and sixties because they've realised that they've spent decades looking after others, and very little time looking after themselves. This is our time to do just that. Meera agrees: 'It's just about making the most of every single moment. I know everybody has ups and downs but it's about making the most of the small gains and the small wins.'

We may live half our adult life post-menopause, and we have this wonderful opportunity now to make the most of our health, to set ourselves up for the future. So if not now, then when?

Meals

To power up through the years ahead, you need to make good nutrition a priority – there's no way round this. I'm not going to tell you that you need to follow a specific diet – you don't. I'm not going to prescribe a regime to follow – you're a grown-up!

We can feel and see body composition changes during and after the menopause transition. Lower oestrogen levels lead to loss of lean body mass and an increase in fat mass. On average, we lose 0.5 per cent of our lean body mass each year during the menopause transition, and increase fat mass by 1.7 per cent.[16] We have to think about what we're eating in the context of these physiological changes.

Below are broad guidelines – but the most important thing I can tell you as your coach is 'don't sweat the small stuff' when it comes to post-menopausal nutrition. Too many of my clients worry about whether or not they should be drinking coconut water, or which brand of tofu they should use, and lose sight of the bigger picture. As women who've faced decades of conditioning from the diet and food industries, we find it hard to make decisions about what's best for us as individuals. Time to take a step back, look at what we're putting on our plates and see what serves us best.

I interviewed menopause nutritionist Jackie Lynch for this section. She's the author of *The Happy Menopause* and presenter of the podcast of the same name. Find her at www. well-well-well.co.uk and @wellwellwelluk on Instagram.

She's in her own power decade and told me: 'I really like being a woman in my fifties. I am conscious that I have to work at it. I have to exercise more, and smarter, than I ever have done before. I have to think much more carefully about what I eat than I did. But the sense of being a woman who has lived, and who has experience, makes me feel much more confident in myself.'

TEN WAYS TO POWER UP YOUR MEALS

1. Lean into Vegetables and Fruit

We need to fill our plates with brightly coloured fruit and vegetables at each meal. It's not rocket science, I know, but my clients make big shifts when they start meal planning with the vegetables first. We tend to think about the protein (meat, fish, cheese, beans etc.) and carbohydrates (bread, rice, pasta) in our meals with vegetables being an afterthought. I urge you to start with the veg, the more brightly coloured the better. These colours come from anti-inflammatory anti-oxidants and are associated with good health and longevity, and a marked reduction in the risk of many of the conditions we want to avoid in the power decade and beyond: ovarian and breast cancer, sarcopenia (muscle wastage), osteopenia and osteoporosis, dementia, metabolic syndrome, even wrinkles. 'Eat the rainbow' has become somewhat of a cliché, but my clients find when they consume plenty of brightly coloured vegetables and fruit, they feel noticeable benefits.

POWER COACHING QUESTION: What's stopping you putting vegetables and fruit first? Habit? Resistant families? Spend some time considering how you can work through these issues.

2. Carbs with Benefits

Carbohydrates – the starchy parts of our meal – have been unfairly demonised in recent years. There's a huge distinction between highly refined, ultra-processed, sugar-laden carbs, and nutrient-dense whole grains, beans and fibrous vegetables that come with a whole host of benefits. We need small amounts (Jackie suggests a fist-sized portion) of starchy foods with each meal. Ask yourself what added benefits your carb choice brings – ideally it comes with fibre plus a little something extra. For example, a sweet potato also brings the antioxidant benefits of carotenoids, which have been linked to better eye and brain health,[17] brown rice has fibre plus B vitamins, green vegetables bring fibre and powerful anti-oxidants to the table.

POWER COACHING QUESTION: How reliant are you on highly processed carbohydrate-rich foods like biscuits, cakes and white pasta? What could you swap in instead?

3. Sugar is Not So Sweet

Sugar, and other refined carbohydrates like white flour, are not our friends. They bring nothing to the party, nutritionally, and send us on a blood sugar rollercoaster just at a time when we've lost the oestrogen that helps keep blood sugar stable (see page 24 for more on this). Jackie urges us to balance blood sugar with enough complex carbohydrates and protein, and to seek out naturally sweet fruits to deliver sweetness without the sugar hit. I know from my own experience, and that of my clients, that three things help us kick sugar to the kerb:

- Making sure that we're eating proper nutritious meals with enough protein and fat so that we feel properly satiated after a meal.
- Understanding the science of sugar's impact on our bodies post-menopause – knowing the damage it wreaks is a strong motivator.
- Finding ways to nourish ourselves that don't involve food. My clients find that prioritising time for themselves, be that reading, relaxing, walking – even Morris dancing! – can help them step away from using sugar for comfort.

POWER COACHING QUESTION: What's driving your cravings? How else could you nourish yourself?

4. How Menopause Has Impacted your Gut . . . and What To Do About It

Our microbiome, the teeming population of bacteria, fungi and viruses that populate our intestines, plays a vital role in disease prevention, longevity and both metabolic and mental health. It's also a key part of the process that regulates weight gain and fat stores. So is oestrogen. And oestrogen also supports good bacteria in the gut. A poorly functioning gut, with an oversupply of bad bacteria, struggles to manage carbohydrate metabolism. This is another link in the chain that creates weight gain post-menopause. Oestrogen and the gut microbiome work together to maintain the integrity of the gut barrier – the single-cell-thick lining that prevents food particles and bacteria entering the bloodstream and causing inflammation. A permeable gut lining is also linked to weight gain and inflammation. Jackie explains, 'The gut is where it all starts. If the gut's not right, ultimately everything else will go wrong as you're not able to absorb vital nutrients correctly.'

As oestrogen declines, we need to do the work ourselves to look after our good gut bacteria and protect our intestinal lining. This means two things – one is introducing healthy new friends to our existing microbiota, in the form of probiotic-rich fermented foods like live natural yogurt, kefir, kimchi and kombucha – or a probiotic supplement if you have histamine sensitivity. The second is to make sure that we're giving our 'team gut' plenty of fibrous foods to ferment. Microbiota 'feed' by fermenting fibrous vegetables and fruits. This process creates short-chain fatty acids that help maintain the structure of our gut wall, making it less likely to 'leak' inflammatory substances into our bodies. Make sure you're getting plenty of the probiotic foods your microbiota like to ferment for their own nourishment: oats, Jerusalem artichokes, cooked and cooled potatoes, almonds, apples, chickpeas, berries, flax and chia seeds, bananas, onions, asparagus, broccoli and kale.

POWER COACHING QUESTION: How can you prioritise your gut health? What simple actions could you take to make a difference?

5. Intermittent Fasting, Yes or No?

I've got to be honest here and say that I'm a big fan of intermittent fasting (a broad term that refers to many different approaches to fasting) to increase longevity and reduce dementia risk. Research has also linked it to weight loss[18] and better glucose management in diabetic patients.[19] The pattern I follow is called time-restricted eating and involves an eating 'window' and a fasting 'window' across a twenty-four-hour period. So that can be a late breakfast, an early dinner or something in between. My eating window is usually about ten hours, or slightly less. It works for me and many of my clients. It doesn't work if you have a history of disordered eating, or low BMI. And for someone still deep in the menopause transition, with intense symptoms, restricting eating times may increase cortisol and make them worse. If that's you, skipping breakfast, rather than starting the day with a filling meal including protein, healthy fats and fibre, isn't going to make you feel any better. I would, however, urge everyone to allow themselves enough time to fully digest dinner before bed. Going to bed on a full stomach impacts our sleep as our bodies pump out insulin to manage glucose, rather than melatonin to aid sleep. Try to finish eating three hours before bed.

Jackie isn't a fan of the '5:2' type of fasting (eat normally for five days a week; restrict calories to about 500 per day for two days), but, like me, recommends time-restricted eating, such as the 16:8 (fast sixteen hours a day; eat in an eight-hour window). She says, 'What I like about it is that you can eat really good, blood-sugar-balancing meals within that. And it keeps things balanced, while taking pressure off the gut. Of course, it doesn't work for everyone, but I think for a lot of us, the 16:8 schedule can be very beneficial.'

POWER COACHING QUESTION: When do you give your body a chance to rest and digest?

6. Low Stomach Acid

The acid in our stomachs – hydrochloric acid (HCL) – helps break down food, aid nutrient absorption and kill off bad bacteria. But levels decline with age, plus oestrogen has a role to play in stomach acid production, so, post-menopause, we may not have enough. Jackie explains, 'If you don't have enough stomach acid you get that feeling of being full very quickly and you may get particles of undigested food moving into the small intestine, causing a lot of bloating, inflammation and discomfort.' At the same time, we may find our oesophagus not working as well as it used to, so we get acid reflux and are prescribed antacids (proton pump inhibitors). They in turn lower stomach acid further. Jackie suggests, 'Try apple cider vinegar, diluted in water, which artificially replaces a little bit of acid before a meal. Bitter herbs can help too, something like chicory. But people who already have acid reflux or a hiatus hernia need to avoid adding more acid.'

POWER COACHING QUESTION: Do you feel bloated? Discomfort after eating? Low stomach acid may be the answer. Try to support your digestion with apple cider vinegar or bitter herbs (unless you have reflux) and talk to your doctor if the issue doesn't resolve.

7. Phytoestrogens

Phyto means plants, and oestrogen . . . well, you know that bit. Put them together and you get naturally occurring compounds that mimic the effects of the hormone in our bodies. These compounds aren't without controversy, and it seems that they have more impact on pre-menopausal and peri-menopausal hormones than on post-menopausal health.[20] Having said that, all foods rich in phytoestrogens also bring other health benefits. Flax seeds, for example, are extremely rich sources of a form of phytoestrogens called lignans, which have been linked to reduced breast-cancer risk in post-menopausal women.[21] Soy beans – usually eaten as tofu, tempeh or edamame – have high levels of isoflavones, also linked to decreased cancer risk. Dried fruit, sesame seeds, garlic, berries, wheat bran and cruciferous vegetables are all good sources too. Jackie tells her clients, 'You have nothing to lose by adding a tablespoon or two of phytoestrogen-rich foods to your diet each day, even if the research is a bit inconclusive. I see in clinic that it can make quite a significant difference to hot flushes.'

POWER COACHING QUESTION: Are you aware of the power of plants to manage oestrogen receptors?

8. Medi Diet

Jackie recommends the Mediterranean diet for its anti-inflammatory properties, which will help to alleviate aching joints, preserve muscle and play a key role in heart health – our hearts being the most important muscle of all. The dietary pattern of traditional Mediterranean communities has also been strongly associated with lower risk of the health issues we want to avoid in our power decade and beyond. It's heavy on vegetables, fruits, whole grains, legumes (beans and pulses), unprocessed oils – particularly olive oil – and includes some fish, eggs and meat. A 2022 study of post-menopausal women in their fifties and sixties looked at the correlation between adherence to the Mediterranean diet and persistent menopause symptoms. It found that those who ate more legumes and pulses had fewer of the physical symptoms of menopause, and those who consumed more olive oil had fewer psychological symptoms.[22] As always, correlation doesn't equal causation, but the results are worth noting. The Mediterranean diet has also been linked to higher bone mass and muscle mass in post-menopausal women,[23] two of the key health issues facing us in our power decade.

POWER COACHING QUESTION: Can you make it Medi? The efficacy of this eating pattern has been extremely well researched in relation to menopause, longevity and all-round good health.

9. Power Up with Protein

We need more, not less, protein as we age because a) our muscles are less able to make use of the protein we consume, and b) we tend to have less muscle to do that work as lean muscle mass declines after the menopause transition (see page 212 for more on increasing muscle mass). This doesn't mean supplementing with protein powder: it means ensuring that we get at least the recommended daily allowance of protein – between 0.8g and 1.2g of protein per kilo of lean body mass* per day – from our regular diet. Many of my clients find, when they work out this equation, they're a long way off. Those who eat very little, or no, animal products find it more difficult to get adequate protein. Not impossible, but more difficult. Meat, fish, eggs and dairy are firmly part of my weekly diet. Non-animal sources include beans, lentils and pulses, soya and tofu, and nuts and seeds.

Jackie is evangelical about protein, finding in clinic that very few women are getting enough. 'Men just seem to instinctively eat it, but women might just have a bit with their evening meal,' she explains. 'And it's not enough because we really need to give our bodies, particularly our bones, the strength they need. And that comes from protein. So many women complain that their hair is thin or their nails are weak. And yes, oestrogen could be a part of that. But are they giving their bodies the tools for the job? Forget about oestrogen for a second; are you getting enough protein? Ask yourself that at every meal and snack.'

---

* What your body weight should be if you were in a healthy BMI range for your height.

If we get our protein from animal sources, we're more likely to be getting a supply of good-quality iron too. When we lose oestrogen, our iron absorption is downregulated, leaving us more vulnerable to anaemia. We need less iron post-menopause (as, for obvious reasons, we're not bleeding so much) but low levels can cause fatigue and headaches. If you're concerned, ask your doctor to check your iron levels.

POWER COACHING QUESTION: Do the equation yourself and evaluate the result – are you getting enough protein? It should be part of every meal.

10. Fat is Your Friend

We're a generation of women who were raised to believe that fat makes us fat, and we should shun it at every opportunity. Many of my clients are triggered simply by the word, telling me that it's not for them, and they'll really struggle to work it into their diets. But we persevere in our coaching sessions because fat is so vitally important to our health as we age. It supports our brain, lubricates our joints and builds healthy cell walls, among many other roles. Fatty fish, such as salmon, sardines and mackerel, provide the omega-3 fatty acids vital for brain health. What else goes on the 'good fat' list? Olive oil, avocados, nuts and seeds – all sources of unprocessed, unsaturated fats. The fats to avoid are the ones that are highly processed, like trans fats and vegetable oils. And the saturated fats found in butter and cheese? Yes, in moderation and the best quality you can get your hands on. Jackie explains, 'Let's not demonise saturated fat, because it's used to create sex hormones. Whether we're on HRT or not, post-menopause we need these hormones. Just making sure we're getting 20–25g of saturated fat daily is important, but it needs to be the good-quality saturated fat: eggs, grass-fed beef, maybe coconut oil. It's one of the building blocks of cholesterol, which, despite the bad press, is the stuff of life. That's what we're made of, really.'

POWER COACHING QUESTION: What are your feelings on fat? Where does that narrative come from – is it rooted in outdated 'fat makes us fat' ideas?

PUTTING IT ALL TOGETHER: WHAT DOES EATING IN THE POWER DECADE LOOK LIKE?

Eating for the post-menopause decade, day in and day out, looks like a plant-forward, fibre-packed diet, with enough protein for our needs and enough healthy fats to keep us feeling full and to lubricate our bodies and brains. I get my clients to imagine a lovely big bowl of food that's going to nourish them and support their health. We line the base of the bowl with lots of leafy greens – spinach, kale, robust salads leaves or rocket. Then we layer in some extra nutrients, carbohydrate and fibre in the form of brightly coloured vegetables: sweet potato, fresh corn, red peppers, red onions, tomatoes. Bonus points for fermented vegetables here like kimchi or sauerkraut. Drizzle over an olive-oil dressing to add healthy fats and aid the digestion of all the nutrients in the veg. Pile in some protein – a piece of salmon, boiled eggs, chicken, some cheese. And top with something for extra flavour – walnuts, almonds, olives. Finish with a square of dark chocolate or some berries. Sounds good, doesn't it?

Jackie reminds us to focus on the enjoyment of eating too, saying, 'Ultimately, if you eat more mindfully, you'll digest better and you'll stop eating when you're ready, rather than hoovering it up. We don't want to take the joy out of food.'

ALCOHOL

I often work with women for whom alcohol has become a friend, there at moments of stress, to help them unwind at the end of the day. One client told me that wine filled the gaps in her life, and for her that meant a bottle of wine a night, most nights. Slowly we unpicked how alcohol had become such an important part of her life, and filled it with more meaningful activities. Alcohol has been linked to worse hot flushes, lower bone density, cognitive decline, sleep disruption, dehydration and mental health issues. None of which we want in our power decade.

Do you have to give up completely? I haven't. But I'm super-aware of how much I drink, enjoying the occasional glass of wine or fizz but always making sure I stay below seven units of alcohol (about three glasses of wine) a week. And I stay hydrated with lots of filtered water and herbal teas.

When my clients cut down on wine, they find it's the early-evening, pre-dinner glass (or two) they miss the most. We introduce 'swaps and swerves' – non-alcoholic drinks that fill the gap without the booze. I love kombucha, but there are so many great non-alcoholic drinks available on the market now. And I'm forever indebted to the client who introduced me to her favourite aperitif – a couple of teaspoons of apple cider vinegar in a glass of sparkling water with ice and a slice of lemon. Great for gut health, stomach acid levels, hydration – and it's cheap!

P.S. Don't forget to stay hydrated! Water is our friend, and thirst cues decline with age.

POWER COACHING QUESTION: Ask yourself what role alcohol plays in your life. What gaps is it filling? How else could you fill those gaps?

Movement

We didn't really need a study to tell us this, but research has shown women become more sedentary during the menopause transition, and then remain on a plateau of low energy expenditure afterwards.[24] It's not surprising because nothing makes us less likely to want to move than menopause – aches and pains, hot flushes, weight gain and tiredness aren't experiences that drive us straight to the gym for an intense workout. But, conversely, nothing makes us need movement MORE than menopause. All those symptoms can be alleviated (to some extent, at least) by movement.

There may also be profound physiological reasons we become more sedentary in our fifties. Fascinating research on mice has found that, when deprived of oestrogen, they simply don't move as much.[25] The brain activity that jumpstarts movement just didn't happen when oestrogen wasn't present. Of course, we move in different ways to mice, but we share many of the same genes and similar hormonal activity. Could it be that oestrogen tells our brains to get us moving?

Add to these physiological changes the huge number of barriers to exercise for older women and the end result is a population of women in their fifties and sixties not moving much at all, and losing muscle each year. Oestrogen protects muscle stem cells:[26] once that declines, it's much harder for our muscles to rebuild and repair without some work on our part. It's movement which will replace that much-needed muscle, keep our bones strong, our hearts healthy and help us manage weight gain.

And let's not forget the many mental benefits of exercise – it can alleviate low moods, stress and sleeplessness. Nothing will put the power into our power decade more than movement, in all its forms.

In one of the Power Women sections on page 46, you'll find an interview with the inspiring Jacqueline Hooton of the wildly popular Instagram account @hergardengym. Jacqueline's been a fitness trainer all her life, and pushes back against ageist narratives in the media which build an expectation that our health will deteriorate. She explains, 'That has direct implications for people actually taking action and understanding what they can do to support their health and wellbeing. If we internalise the idea that our forties onwards is going to be a time of decline, we're not going to put the work in to look after ourselves.' Be aware of your own thoughts on this: do you *expect* post-menopause to be a time of decline? Where's that narrative coming from?

The other narrative we need to change is that exercise is for weight loss. We may have spent decades exercising to burn calories: memorising the stats that told us that twenty minutes on the treadmill would 'burn off' half a doughnut, or whatever. The end result is that the importance of fitness for health has been ignored. Jacqueline explains, 'I think so many women have a bad relationship with fitness because it's always been about weight loss. And that's never turned out right for them, so they've ended up with a bad relationship with their body. Whereas if we bring it back to the health conversation and we help people get stronger, and feel more physically able, they feel so much better about fitness.'

I also interviewed women's health physio and co-founder of Menopause Movement, Christien Bird, for this section. Find her at whitehartclinic.co.uk, menopausemovement.co, @christienbirdphysio and @menopausemovement. She believes movement and muscles are our best friend in menopause. When we spoke, she'd just returned – aged fifty-nine – from Slovakia, where she was part of the team representing GB in the Aquathlon World Championships. And while that level of movement is a bit daunting for many, it's certainly inspiring!

As always, seek expert advice, make sure you have the right kit and always warm up and warm down appropriately when you exercise.

TEN WAYS TO POWER UP YOUR MOVEMENT

1. Your Mindset on Movement

My clients range from exercise experts and marathon runners to those for whom a brisk walk is exhausting. Most are somewhere in between, wondering where the fitness of their younger years has gone and how to work movement into busy lives. The first thing we work on is what's doable and realistic for them. There's no point me telling someone who hasn't exercised for years to get to the gym every day, but I can get her to start walking. And I can nudge a relatively fit woman into getting her bike repaired when it's fallen into disuse, or suggest that the marathon runner works some stretching into her week. Where do you fit in here? And how do you feel about the level of movement in your life? If you're not exercising, can you evaluate why?

Christien believes shame plays a role. She told me, 'It breaks my heart that the main barrier for many women not going to a gym or exercise facility is shame: shame about how they look, that they're not fit enough, that they might be too fat, you name it. All those shame issues are there.' Her solution to this? 'Do things with a buddy. Make it a social connection and start moving together. If you do it with someone else, at least you can laugh about it!'

POWER COACHING QUESTION: Is your barrier to exercise your mindset? Ask yourself what you want to be fit for.

2. Movement All Day, Every Day

Exercise can be a daunting and off-putting word, with its connotations of vigorous workouts, Lycra and PE lessons. I'm using the word 'movement' in this chapter because that's what we need: climbing stairs, running for the bus, carrying shopping bags, walking round the block. It's all movement and it all counts. Our world is increasingly sedentary and convenient; we have gadgets to clean (thank goodness!), our shopping can be delivered, we've probably got a car to drive. And chances are we're chained to a desk for longer than ever each day. All these things mean we're moving less than our foremothers. Scientists talk about 'non-exercise activity thermogenesis' (NEAT)[27] – the way we use energy other than for basic metabolic tasks like breathing and digestion, or exercise. NEAT happens when we undertake other forms of movement as we go about our daily activities – such as walking, standing or even fidgeting – and may be the most important activity we do each day.

POWER COACHING QUESTION: How 'NEAT' are you? How often do you move throughout the day?

3. Walking, and Walking Faster

The movement gods have given a gift to those of us who are post-menopausal and it's called walking. We're designed to do it, it's free, usually easy and it's incredibly good for us. The classic exhortation is 10,000 steps a day but that's a large and sometimes daunting number. Luckily, research published in autumn 2022 gives us a more nuanced view.[28] Researchers found that every 2,000 steps walked lowered the risk of premature death incrementally by between 8 per cent and 11 per cent. There was a correlation between the number of daily steps and reduced risk of dementia, heart disease and cancer way before the magic 10,000 steps: the risk of dementia was reduced by 25 per cent at as low as 3,800 steps a day. The study also found that increasing the pace of walking benefits all those outcomes, and can make fewer steps count significantly more. If 10,000 steps seems daunting or too time-consuming, picking up the pace can make all the difference.

POWER COACHING QUESTION: If you track your steps, can you walk more than your annual daily average today? It's a simple way to keep increasing your daily step count.

4. HIIT (High-Intensity Interval Training) and Cardio

What's your response to the idea of high-intensity training? 'Never in a million years' or 'Bring it!'? At its most basic level, HIIT is a way of getting out of breath for a short time, then having a period of lower-intensity exercise or rest. This could be gently pedalling on an exercise bike, then speeding up for twenty seconds before going back to a gentler pace. It's a fast, efficient way to gain the cardiovascular benefits of exercise without spending hours pounding a treadmill.

Now, you might love cardio exercise – if running, tennis, or any sport for that matter, is your jam, enjoy every moment of it. But intense exercise may not be the best thing for us after the menopause transition. Some boot-camp-style exercises, or slogging away on a cross-trainer, can increase the stress hormone cortisol (which in turn can increase fat storage around our mid-section) and put pressure on joints. Getting a bit breathless and sweaty is life-enhancing; pounding away causing ourselves stress and pain isn't. Jacqueline adds, 'Women often hate cardiovascular training because it's associated with pain. It's something they might have done a lot to try to lose weight and that never worked. So instead you could try a brisk walk, which can support heart health, or something else you like, such as swimming, or cycling with older children.'

For Christien, however, it's clear that most of the women she sees aren't exercising enough. 'Through the menopause, we lose lean muscle mass and we lose our lung capacity, our VO2 max. We need to work beyond our comfort zone – wherever that is – because it's in the discomfort where you get the benefits.'

POWER COACHING QUESTION: What does it take for you to get breathless? How often do you do that?

5. Making Muscle and Bone: Strength Training

If I had to name one magic bullet for thriving in the power decade, it would be strength training. Our muscle mass and bone density decline post-menopause once we lose that protective cloak of oestrogen and become more sedentary. Along with falling oestrogen, we experience a decline in growth hormone concentrations after menopause, which is also linked to decreased muscle mass. Less muscle means fewer ways to burn up glucose and an increased risk of insulin resistance. Not to mention the fact that less muscle makes us more vulnerable to falls. This is a perfect example of Mother Nature giving us a little shove and telling us to get on with looking after ourselves: we need to keep building muscle throughout our lives.

'I would absolutely prioritise strength training over anything else,' says Jacqueline. It lowers our chance of dying from all causes, increases our metabolism, helps stabilise glucose, improves balance and bones, keeps us mobile and has a huge impact on mental wellbeing. Jacqueline sees it helping her clients build self-esteem. What's not to love? Oh, the training bit. But strength training doesn't have to mean heaving dumbbells around in a sweaty gym (although that's cool) – it can be weight machines, bodyweight classes, resistance bands, reformer Pilates, hand weights, kettlebells – anything that loads your muscles to the point of tiredness, rather than exhaustion. Christien urges us to do what puts a smile on our faces, asking, 'What do you like? I think if people don't like gyms, don't go to the gym because it could be miserable.'

POWER COACHING QUESTION: What are you doing to load your muscles?

6. Stretching Mind and Body

When I talk to my clients about how they see their future health, maintaining mobility is one of the key issues they always reference. To do that we need to keep flexible, preserving our range of motion for as long as we can. Jacqueline reminds us of the importance of retaining movement in the joints 'so we can do those things like put something into a cupboard, or get in and out of a car: all those things which we know can go wrong the older we get'.

Yoga has been found to reduce hot flushes and improve quality of life among women with an average age of fifty-five,[29] while other research has found it improves sleep and lowers stress. Yoga, Pilates and tai chi are all wonderful ways to connect body and mind, and to stretch out muscles and joints that may stiffen in our power decade. But we don't have to seek out an organised class to reap the benefits of stretching: a simple stretch routine at our desk, or when we wake up in the morning, can make all the difference. If you don't know where to start, try a forward fold, which increases blood flow to the pelvic region and the brain, as well as stretching out the back and thighs. Stand in a comfortable position with your feet firmly planted on the ground and knees slightly bent. Roll your spine down so your head and arms hang down and relax. Take a couple of breaths, then gently roll up again, stacking your vertebrae so your head comes up last.

POWER COACHING QUESTION: When are you going to stretch? How about now?

7. Balance and Posture

If we are to avoid the falls that can plague women in older age, we need to work on balance and posture in the power decade. Around the age of sixty seems to be the point at which balance declines, and an inability to stand on one leg for ten seconds is linked to higher mortality. Menopause itself can impact balance, as oestrogen loss may affect the inner ear for some. Yoga, Pilates and tai chi-type exercises all help with balance and posture, or, again, you can do simple exercises at home that will help. The classic is standing on one leg while you brush your teeth, but you could also try brushing your teeth standing against a wall, with your shoulders and head touching the wall, to improve postural alignment. And how about trying to stand on one leg while shutting your eyes – how long can you remain stable for? The ideal for the over-fifties is at least eight seconds. With eyes open it should be more than forty seconds. Make sure you've got something to catch hold of if you start to wobble!

POWER COACHING QUESTION: Can you commit to working on your balance and posture? What would it take for you to do that? There's more on this on page 226.

8. Get Outside

Daylight is the secret sauce that enhances the benefits of every movement we make. Morning light, every morning, is a non-negotiable for me because it sets our circadian rhythms, kickstarting the cycle that makes us alert first thing and sleepy in the evening. A ten-minute stroll is all it takes to reap the benefits, while also reducing stress and working movement into our day. It can provide vital vitamin D too (when the sun is high enough in the sky). Cold exposure isn't for everyone, but it has convincing health benefits. It could be cold-water swimming, a cold shower or just a walk in cold weather. Benefits include blood glucose stabilisation, better immunity and improved mood.

POWER COACHING QUESTION: How much daylight do you really see?

9. You and Your Pelvic Floor

There are more oestrogen receptors in our vaginal muscles, pelvic floor and bladder than anywhere else in the body. When oestrogen declines, the muscles of these areas are more impacted than any other tissue: they weaken and thin.

The result is a risk of bladder problems and pain. 'The good news,' Christien explains, 'is that this is incredibly easy to treat with topical vaginal oestrogen. Some women will have enough oestrogen, but most women will need a little bit of topical oestrogen combined with pelvic floor muscle training.' See page 128 for more on this.

So, how do you train these muscles, in order to help prevent problems in the first place? When we think about pelvic floor exercises, we usually think about 'kegels', where we squeeze and hold the 3D mesh of muscles that supports our urethra, vagina and colon. Simple exercises include:

- Squeeze the muscles around your back passage, vagina and urethra as if you're trying to stop yourself peeing. Feel the internal squeeze and lift. Then fully relax the muscles before doing it again.
- Do ten slow squeezes of ten seconds each, then ten fast one-second squeezes. Make sure you fully relax between each one. There's more on the Squeezy app, which will also send daily reminders to squeeze!
- Moving beyond the squeeze, we need to remember that it's not really a pelvic floor at all, it's a diaphragm, which rises and falls with each breath just like the diaphragm under our ribs. The pelvic diaphragm supports the downward movement of our internal organs as we breathe. So proper deep rhythmic breathing helps to gently contract and release the pelvic muscles.

- Muscles of the pelvic floor attach to the femur, so actions that work the thighs, like squats and lunges, also work the pelvic floor. As we release from these movements, we're working against gravity, activating the pelvic muscles. We need to be careful that we're not over-stressing the pelvic floor with these exercises, however, so always work within your capacity.

If you're still struggling with pelvic health problems, talk to your GP and ask to be referred to a women's health physio. Under NICE guidelines, it's mandatory for your doctor to refer you if you have such issues, so don't be afraid to ask.

POWER COACHING QUESTION: Are you prioritising the importance of working on your pelvic floor post-menopause?

10. Rest

Rest is, of course, the opposite of movement, but I think of it as the missing piece of the puzzle when it comes to good health! We are so conditioned to be 'on' all the time: there's always another thing to do, a box set to watch, a chore to finish, work to complete. We don't allow ourselves time to rest and replenish our energy levels. If we're trying to get stronger, strength training creates micro-tears in our muscle, which need to heal and repair to build new muscle. This only happens when we're resting, not when we're exercising.

Resting doesn't have to mean going to bed or staring out of the window. Using our downtime wisely can mean walking in nature, reading a book, meditation or a mindfulness practice: whatever feels right for us.

POWER COACHING QUESTION: What's holding you back from working rest into your life? My clients find it hard to schedule fifteen minutes to do nothing, but try it!

PUTTING IT ALL TOGETHER: WHAT DOES MOVING IN THE POWER DECADE LOOK LIKE?

If I could urge you to do one thing, it would be to do the thing you *can* do. And then do it a little harder, or faster, or longer. Start there. Forget the idea that you have to be in a gym to exercise. One of my clients decided a treadmill in her garage was the thing for her and does fast incline walking intervals while watching her favourite TV shows; another – in her mid-seventies – decided she liked the look of that Joe Wicks and works out to his videos at home.

Think about variety – when are you building muscle? What's helping you stretch? How do you get your heart pumping? It's this variety of movement that will help you power up.

INJURY AND PAIN

One of the key reasons I find my clients aren't moving is fear of injury and pain. If we've got out of the habit of exercise, fear can be a real barrier. But, as Christien says, it's not safe NOT to exercise. We'll get injured walking downstairs, or getting off the sofa, or possibly just standing still if we don't put the work in to maintain bone density and muscle mass. Christien points out, 'Exercise is anti-inflammatory, so it helps reduce pain from joint inflammation. We have this pain anyway, so why not find a way to exercise that helps?'

Christien adds, 'I think because we're alive and because we've got spines and we've got joints, we will get injured. That's the simple truth. I spend a lot of time explaining that to women and telling them we just have to find out what works. It's important to remember we don't need to be pain-free all the time. A little bit of pain is fine, in fact it's probably quite good for us. But at the same time, you obviously don't want to overdo it and injure yourself more. It's about getting that balance right and giving women confidence that they can move.'

Power Women: Jo McEwan and Ann Stephens, Positive Pause

When I began looking after my own health, Jo, 58, and Ann, 60, were the first women I came across who were talking about menopause in an open and accessible way. They set up Positive Pause to share supportive and constructive advice about midlife, menopause and beyond. More recently, they've developed the platform Menopause Movement with women's health physio Christien Bird, an online training and community platform for health and fitness professionals. So not only are they helping other women, they've also set up two successful businesses in their fifties.

For Jo and Ann, as for so many women, the arrival of perimenopausal symptoms was a shock. Jo explains, 'Nine years ago, aged forty-nine, I went to the doctors for some antibiotics and she asked me how I was feeling. I told her I was a bit tired, my hair was getting thin, and she said, 'Well, you are perimenopausal.' I knew what menopause was, but I'd never heard the word perimenopausal. I went straight onto Google and from everything I read it made me feel I was on a Stannah stairlift to old age! I kept asking friends, like Ann, "How can we not know about this? We know how to get our kids into school, how to insure a car; how can we not know about this?" I said I felt like setting up a website. There was nothing positive or empowering to support us. And Ann's response was, "Right, let's do it."'

Like Jo, Ann had little understanding of the word perimenopause and her symptoms were quite different. 'I was still having periods, I never had hot flushes and I had only associated menopause with women whose periods had stopped and who had hot flushes. Neither of those things were happening to me but I was having a complete psychological breakdown. I'm self-employed and I was making mistakes, suffering brain fog, having panic attacks, bursting into tears, terrified to speak on the phone. When Jo mentioned perimenopause, I joined the dots and thought, it's my hormones, not me! I was so shocked there wasn't something out there to help, so when Jo mentioned creating our website I said, "If you're really serious, I'm in."'

From those early conversations came two fabulous platforms that support women in midlife: a real personal achievement for them both. Jo explains, 'I've probably learned more since I've been doing this than at any other time in my life in terms of new skills and new information. I think sometimes we're not proud enough of what we've achieved: if you'd asked me five years ago if I'd be addressing big charities and multi-national corporations on menopause, I'd have said, "Don't be ridiculous!"'

Ann adds, 'As women we get so used to multitasking, looking after everyone else and making sure everyone's life is in order. You're never looking at yourself. And I think there's a freedom when the kids fly the nest, and you suddenly have time for yourself and to think about the type of work you want to do. Work gives you a lot of freedom as you get older. I've got so many friends who are retiring, and I don't want to contemplate that. I love what I do; there's never two days the same. There's always something new to learn or someone new to talk to.'

The knock-on effect of setting up health-related businesses has been an increase in confidence both mentally and physically. Ann says, 'I certainly feel in my body more, more supple, fewer aches and pains. I just feel fit and I feel ten times better than I did in my thirties, forties or fifties. And that's to do with the fact that Positive Pause has made me focus on that. I feel more confident in myself. As a young person, I was always very conscious of what I looked like and what people thought of me. I still care what I look like, but I don't care what people think any more.

'You only have one body and it's up to you to look after it. No one else can do it for you. Of course, there are certain conditions people have no control over, but in terms of menopause you've got to take ownership. I liken it to a car that you have to MOT every year. If you decide to go on a long journey, you don't want it to break down and therefore you've got to look after it. Similarly, you have to look after yourself if you want to live longer.'

Jo adds, 'There's life on the other side of menopause, a different life. You're older, you've wised up and you've hopefully got a lot longer to live. Take control of your life, take some risks, step outside your comfort zone. I know we all have very different opportunities but, fundamentally, if you do the best you can you're going to be a lot happier. Who wants a miserable old age? Let's get it sorted now.'

Find Ann and Jo at Positive Pause, www.positivepause.co.uk and @positivepauseuk on Instagram/Facebook, and Menopause Movement, www.menopausemovement.co and @menopausemovement.

Power Women: Jo Moseley

I found Jo, 58, on social media shortly after Annabel and I founded The Age-Well Project. I've followed Jo's warm-hearted and inspiring journeys – literal and figurative – ever since. She describes herself as a joy encourager, beach cleaner and midlife adventurer. Good health in the great outdoors is at the heart of her own power decade, which has included stand-up paddleboarding across the waterways of England, becoming an award-winning filmmaker and writing a bestselling book, *Stand-Up Paddleboarding in Great Britain: Beautiful Places to Paddleboard in England, Scotland and Wales.*

Jo has spoken openly about how broken she felt by perimenopause, which for her coincided with being a single mum, and both her parents receiving a cancer diagnosis. One day she found herself crying in the biscuit aisle of a supermarket. 'I just burst into tears because I couldn't cope any more. It was just overwhelming and I didn't realise it was the menopause. I was just exhausted, not sleeping, heart palpitations, night sweats, headaches, tinnitus, that awful itchy skin, those joint pains which are difficult to describe. And utter anxiety. I told a friend and she lent me an old rowing machine. I started exercising, and then I started sleeping. That was great because sleep is my big thing, it's so important to me.'

From that very low moment in the supermarket, Jo was able to gradually move forward. 'I joined a gym to exercise more, then, in December of that year, my mum died. I realised that rowing in the gym was helping my grief; it was so much more than just the physicality. I rowed one million metres, and a marathon, to raise money for Macmillan Cancer Support, and I started to believe in myself a bit more. I felt as if I was piecing myself back together. I read books by Brené Brown, who said, "It's your story, it's your ending." I'd spent my whole life being very reactive, supporting other people. I was never on the priority list. It took me a long time, a really, really long time, to believe that another ending was possible, one that I could be proud of.

'I've just done it bit by bit, trying to make changes, trying to put myself on the priority list. I don't have a huge budget, so it's basic, simple stuff. Walking, paddleboarding, swimming – it's about tiny steps and battling the voice that says, "Put everyone else first."

'Life is short and precious. If you have a chance of some joy, and making a difference, then you should try and do that. I started my little films and my podcast and my book by just exploring. With each step I was rebuilding a foundation of confidence. I'd think, "Well, you did *that* and it went OK, maybe you could do *this* now." I create massive goals for myself and then I think I've just got to take it inch by inch, step by step.

'Back when everything was crumbling around me, I read an Albert Camus quote: "In the depths of winter, I finally learned that within me there lay an invincible summer." I remember looking at it, thinking, "I have no summer within me." But maybe I could find that summer. So being with my family, paddleboarding, swimming, my creative projects – they're all about finding that summer. It's about being able to say, "It's quite sunny in my heart."

'I want to encourage people to understand that they're worth it, and that their goals and dreams are worth pursuing. Have that internal conversation with yourself, take the time and the mental space to do that – carve out that time for yourself.'

I asked Jo how she looks after herself now. 'I know I can't wing it. I need regular bedtimes, getting outside and exercise otherwise there's stress when I take too much on and my anxiety gets worse. I do feel like I've had this massive creative burst and now I need to have a period of nourishment so I can recalibrate and regenerate. I've got myself through the menopause and I know I'm OK. I need to have boundaries around my time, and I've learned not to push myself to the edge. I see having purpose as a health issue. My beach cleans, giving talks, writing books and articles, seeing friends – they all give me purpose. I did a talk recently and I took copies of my book to sell, and I was looking at it, thinking, "Wow, that's my name on there!" Sometimes I have to remind myself that I did that.'

When Jo looks back to where she was ten years ago, it's hard to imagine how far she's come. 'In my twenties, I went diving to look for hammerhead sharks in the Philippines, and I didn't think anything of it. By my forties I was scared to go to Sainsbury's after dark. I felt ground down, scared of the world. I'm not saying I'd go diving to look for hammerheads again now, but I've re-found that lost courage. Outwardly, I don't look very different, but I think the landscape within me is very different. And, to me, that is the key. That's the summer. And if I can keep that summer alive into my golden years, it'll be quite a sunny time.'

Find Jo at jomoseley.com and @jomoseley on Instagram and Twitter.

SECTION 3

POWER UP BODY AND MIND TO FEEL YOUR BEST RIGHT NOW

Introduction

There are as many post-menopausal experiences as there are post-menopausal women on the planet – and there are more than one billion of us! I've talked to many hundreds of women while writing this book and all have a very different experience in their fifties and sixties. There's no right or wrong way to go through the power decade. But some experiences are broadly shared.

A lot of women continue to experience menopausal symptoms, particularly disrupted sleep, hot flushes, night sweats and brain fog. Some find relief in HRT. Genitourinary symptoms can be particularly distressing and can appear many years after the final menstrual period. Some women, on the other hand, feel great – unyoked from the endless rolling menstrual cycle and years of perimenopausal symptoms.

Mentally and emotionally, responses are very varied too. This stage of life can bring loss, workplace difficulties and heavy caring burdens. It may be a time when we face up to our own mortality, and society's ambivalence towards ageing women. But it can also be a period of great freedom, of renewal and of expansion. It can be a time when we start to feel 'ourselves' again.

Most often, I believe, how we feel right now is a complex combination of all these factors – some noticeable physical issues combined with a strong desire to nurture ourselves to the best possible health; anxiety about our role in the world coupled with excitement about a new stage in life. None of this is easy to navigate, but let me give you a toolkit to get you on your way.

I've divided this section about immediate health issues you may be experiencing into two parts: 'Body' and 'Mind'. Each begins with one key action to focus on – sleep in the 'Body' section, and stress in 'Mind'. We then break down the persistent symptoms of menopause that may stay with you past the final menstrual period, well into your fifties, sixties and beyond.

BODY
Do This First . . . Prioritise Sleep

I meet a lot of women who, post-menopause, are working hard on their health. They're eating well and taking regular exercise. And then I ask them about sleep. 'Oh, *sleep*,' they say. 'I don't sleep well at all.' Sleep is so foundational to good health but often eludes us. There are a few outliers, of course: the women in their fifties who can throw themselves into bed at any time and get a deeply restorative eight hours. But they're few and far between. I'm always surprised – and rather jealous – when I meet one!

When I surveyed followers of The Age-Well Project, those in the fifty-six to sixty-five age bracket reported sleep issues as their worst, and most persistent, symptom post-menopause. This was closely followed by night sweats and brain fog. An unholy trinity of symptoms that all feed into one another. Our sleep is disturbed by our dysfunctional vasomotor system, so the exhaustion we feel the next day exacerbates mood and memory problems. Sound familiar? Around half of women experience sleep disruption in midlife and 30–40 per cent report chronic insomnia by the end of menopause.

To sleep well we need to look at both the internal and external factors keeping us awake. Internal factors could involve stress, anxiety and hormonal issues; external factors relate to the environment in which we're trying to sleep. We need to work on both if we want to sleep well, and commit to making changes. When I talk to clients, I find their sleep issues are often rooted in a belief that they don't deserve to put themselves first. They'll give me a long list of reasons they can't sleep, from wakeful teens to snoring husbands. The power decade is all about reclaiming our time and identity, and that includes finding ways to sleep.

THE LINK BETWEEN SLEEP AND REPRODUCTIVE HORMONES

When we sleep, our bodies and brains go through an incredible process of recovery and rejuvenation: it's as vital to good health as moving and eating. Mental health, cognition, the cardiovascular system, metabolism, immune function and strength are all impacted by the quality of our sleep.

The hormone progesterone is particularly linked to sleep, and it dwindles to nothing during the menopause transition. Progesterone has a calming effect and increases production of a neurotransmitter – a chemical in the brain – called GABA, which helps us sleep by calming neural activity. Lower levels of progesterone, and GABA, can lead to symptoms like anxiety and disturbed sleep, particularly frequent waking.

Oestrogen, the reproductive hormone at the root of so many of the changes of menopause, also helps regulate our body temperature at night, keeping us cool so we're more likely to get restful sleep. Those night sweats? They're the result of fluctuating oestrogen levels causing sudden temperature changes as we sleep.

Add to all this the fact that melatonin, the primary driver of our sleep cycle, is itself a hormone, so is impacted by changing levels of other hormones like oestrogen and progesterone – and all in all, we've got a toxic cocktail of sleep deprivation on our hands.

OTHER CAUSES OF SLEEP ISSUES IN THE POWER DECADE

Ageing: The simple fact of getting older has a strong impact on sleep. Our circadian rhythms, the internal clocks that run our sleep and wake cycles, get knocked out of whack as we age. Over fifty, a second clock starts to develop, at odds with the first, and that impacts our sleep quality. The body creates more 'body clock' genes as age impacts the ones we're born with, but the end result is a system that's out of sync.[30] Anchoring our clocks with regular sleep and wake times can help alleviate this.

Increased stress: Many of us find the years after the menopause transition empowering and exciting. But this is also a period of profound, and sometimes stressful, change. Stress triggers our 'fight or flight' response, meaning that we are 'on' and ready to take action at a moment's notice. When we're stressed our heart rate, blood pressure and blood sugar are elevated, and our autonomic nervous system floods us with the hormones cortisol and adrenaline. None of which is conducive to a good night's sleep.

Insomnia and anxiety: Let's be clear: sleep deprivation and insomnia are two different things. We deprive ourselves of sleep by not spending enough time in bed, by not having an effective routine for sleep, or by sabotaging our body's attempts to get us to sleep. Insomnia, on the other hand, is a clinical disorder, often related to anxiety, resulting in the brain firing up at night, never allowing the body a break from the adrenaline and cortisol needed to keep it awake during the day. Anxiety, stress and depression are some of the most common causes of chronic insomnia. And, of course, having difficulty sleeping can also make those symptoms worse. As you address your sleep habits, you need first to be clear about what's causing problems, if you have them. Do you need to address wider emotional issues that are causing you anxiety? Or are you feeling anxious because of a lack of sleep? The two are often closely intertwined. I would urge you to seek help for anxiety, via your GP.

What's keeping us awake?: The modern world is designed to keep us awake. There's always another episode to binge on Netflix, another email to send, another social media feed to scroll. If we're awake, we're consuming, and – often – that means spending too. That's how the twenty-first-century economy works. Not to mention societal pressures to have everything under control, be busy, be 'on' all the time. Sleep has become an indulgence: it's for wimps. We lionise people who can get by on a few hours' sleep a night and wish we knew their secret. So – AND THIS IS REALLY IMPORTANT – it's not our fault we can't sleep. The world is designed to keep us from sleep – and, as women, we've internalised messages that we should do everything, be the best we can and help everyone, all the time.

POWER UP: SMALL DAILY HABITS TO IMPROVE SLEEP

MINDSET

Do you believe you're a bad sleeper?

Silly question, really, but research has found that one factor that may influence sleep quality as we age is what the scientists called 'sleep-related metacognitive activity', such as our beliefs about sleeping difficulties, and night-time thought-control strategies.[31] What this means is that if we believe we can't sleep and we keep telling ourselves that, we're less likely to be able to sleep; in other words, if our beliefs about sleep are dysfunctional, our sleep will be dysfunctional. We need to upgrade our beliefs around sleep, and integrate small daily habits for better sleep into our lives. When my clients give me a long list of reasons why they *can't* sleep, I ask them to write a list of why they *can*.

Understand that waking in the night is normal

Each night we sleep in cycles, going from light sleep to deep, then a rapid eye movement (REM) phase, in which we're more likely to dream. As we finish a cycle we may wake. And that's OK. It's part of the normal cycle, not necessarily a sign that we're suffering terrible sleeplessness. If we just accept it's part of a cycle, maybe potter to the loo and then get back into bed with the expectation that we're going to fall asleep again, then we're more likely to do just that. It's a simple mindset shift, but my clients find it effective.

Allow yourself to go to bed

We need to break through the idea that we should be 'on' all the time and – wait for it – go to bed! It sounds so simple, doesn't it? But there's a lot to unpack here. It's very easy to self-sabotage our own bedtime, and our sleep. That might be because we're so busy dealing with the needs of others – bosses, family, parents – that we try to carve out some time for ourselves late in the evening rather than go to bed. Psychologists call this 'revenge bedtime procrastination'. The term refers to the idea of 'taking revenge' on a hectic and stressful day by reclaiming time for leisure activities at night, even if that comes at the cost of our own sleep. It creates a vicious cycle of sleep deprivation, more procrastination because we're tired, then more sleep deprivation, and so on. It seems that the less self-determination we get in the day due to a stressful job or other responsibilities, the more we want to reclaim our own time.

Treat sleep like a hobby you're passionate about

Changing our mindset on sleep means giving it the attention, and sometimes investment, it deserves. Invest in the right kit – a good mattress, pillows, eye masks, ear plugs, blackout blinds and curtains have all been shown to improve sleep duration and quality. And dedicate time to it, as you would a favourite hobby. Don't allow yourself that bedtime procrastination – what could be better revenge on a hectic day than a good night's sleep?

Create a wind-down routine

We'll all have a different take on what that might be, but it's about slowing down and starting to get ready for the night ahead. It might include dimming the lights in the house so the brain prepares for sleep, switching off screens, having a bath or a cup of chamomile tea, writing a gratitude list or evening journalling. Experiment and see which is best for you.

Ideas for a gratitude list

This doesn't need to be long and complicated, just enough to help us tune into what we have to be grateful for in life. This practice helps us focus on the joys we have in front of us and cultivates healthy habits. Try filling out this list:

Today I am grateful for . . .

People: _____
Events: _____
Items: _____

If you do wake in the night . . .

Visualise things that make you happy . . .
Try to replace the negative worry loop with mental images of a place that makes you feel happy and calm. This is called imagery distraction. Where's that happy place for you? A beach, on the water, in the woods, a friend's house? Take your mind there rather than to your worries.

. . . And create positive affirmations about sleep
We use affirmations to instil healthy and positive beliefs in ourselves. Creating affirmations around sleep, believing we can sleep, makes a difference. Try:

I am feeling positive about my sleep
I can have a good night's sleep

What can you add?

    I am _____

    I can _____

If that doesn't work, don't lie in bed tossing and turning

Dr Carys Sonnenberg suggests that, if you are struggling to sleep, try having a regular routine: going to bed, and getting up at around the same time every day. 'If you are lying in bed and struggling to sleep, the best thing to do is to get up after about twenty minutes,' she says. 'Try to go to another room, with the lights dimmed, and relax there until you feel tired and then go back to bed. Many people lie in bed tossing and turning. It is helpful to teach your brain that your bed is for sleeping and having sex only, not for worrying and tossing and turning.'

MEALS

Not just what, but when

When we eat before bed is as important as what we eat. We need to allow our bodies to digest properly before we try to sleep, as we're simply not designed to do both things at once. Melatonin, the sleep hormone, runs on the same pathway as insulin, which manages glucose from food. The body can't produce both at once, and will prioritise glucose management over sleep. You know that feeling when you don't sleep well after a late meal? This is why. Try leaving three hours between eating and digestion. When I worked in an office and had a daily commute, I found this difficult, but I did what I could. Two hours to digest before bed is still better than nothing.

What to eat is important too

We all know the kinds of meals that keep us awake, usually something stodgy and sugary. A meal high in refined carbohydrates, which requires lots of insulin to manage, has a far more detrimental impact on our sleep than a meal including quality protein and fibre. That doesn't mean eating steak every night – lots of people find red meat hard to digest as they age – but aim to consume an evening meal that nourishes you rather than sends you on a blood-sugar crash and burn.

Nutrients for good sleep

Many of the foods recommended in the Meals section (see page 196) provide nutrients that help power up sleep. Vitamin B6 helps with the production of melatonin and can be found in sunflower seeds, tuna and wild salmon, avocado, chicken, cooked spinach, bananas, potatoes and whole grains. Magnesium is a key nutrient for sleep and many women are deficient. Find it in almonds, leafy greens, bananas and fish. Vitamin B12 helps to regulate the sleep-wake cycle by keeping our circadian rhythms in sync. Find it in meat, dairy, eggs, fish and shellfish. Vegans need to supplement.

Drinks for sleep

I extol the virtues of a small, strong cup of chamomile tea before bed. Don't have a giant mugful; you'll be up all night going to the loo. Think of it like an espresso, but one that will help you sleep rather than keep you awake. The sedative qualities of chamomile are attributed to apigenin, an antioxidant that binds to receptors in the brain, decreasing anxiety and helping us sleep. Alcohol, on the other hand, isn't our friend at bedtime – or any other time, to be honest. I track my sleep using an Oura ring and I can see that even one small glass of wine makes a difference to the amount of deep sleep I get. Ditto caffeine too late in the day.

Grab foods that make GABA

GABA (gamma-aminobutyric acid) is a neurotransmitter that helps us feel relaxed, and so is linked to better sleep. The body naturally makes GABA in the gut and it functions as part of the gut–brain connection. Beneficial bacteria in the gut, like *Lactobacillus* and *Bifidobacterium*, produce GABA. We can also get it from certain foods like green leafy vegetables, soy beans, mushrooms, tomatoes, buckwheat, peas, brown rice and sweet potatoes.

MOVEMENT

A hot bath or shower

When we sleep, the body experiences a very subtle drop in temperature, just enough to tell the brain that it's sleep time. We can mimic and amplify that effect with a hot bath or shower. As we step out of the hot water into a cool room, our body temperature drops, making the brain think that it's time to wind down. Studies have shown people who do this have better sleep efficiency, which means more of the time they're in bed they're actually asleep.

A physiological sigh

Invented back in the 1930s, this simple breathwork technique can be used to improve both stress and sleep levels, which are so closely linked. It blows carbon dioxide out of your lungs quickly: one aspect of the stress response is having too much CO_2 in the bloodstream and lungs, so blowing off CO_2 rapidly calms the brain and nervous system. Take a long, strong inhale through the nose into the diaphragm, until almost full capacity. Then take one more quick, short burst, getting a little extra air into the lungs. This short top-up breath opens up the alveoli and allows access to the CO_2 they're holding on to. Then take a long, slow exhale through the mouth, to offload that CO_2 build-up. Two or three breaths are enough for a calming effect, or try ten to fifteen to help you sleep.

Exercise

Aerobic exercise helps us sleep, although researchers still aren't completely sure why. People who do around thirty minutes of moderate exercise during the day get better sleep that night, so we don't have to wait long to see the results! It doesn't really matter what it is, as long as it's something you enjoy. Some people find that, if they exercise too close to bedtime, it impacts sleep quality. This may be due to the production of endorphins (feelgood hormones), which make us more alert. Or it may be because exercise raises our body temperature. If you're an evening exerciser, make sure you allow enough time for your body temperature to drop before bed.

Morning, evening and artificial light

Getting daylight on our eyeballs in the morning is one of the best ways of ensuring a good night's sleep in the evening. Seeing blue light in the morning (that doesn't mean the sky has to be blue, just that we're outside) tells our brain that it's morning and it's time to kickstart the circadian rhythms that will make us feel sleepy twelve to fourteen hours later. If our brain doesn't get that signal, it can't fire the starting pistol on our day, so our sleep is likely to be compromised that night. Similarly, if we can get outside as the light fades in the evening, it's a signal to our brain that bedtime is approaching. That's why the blue light from screens is so disruptive to our sleep. Our brains read it as morning light and go into wake-up mode. Switch those screens off at least an hour before bed.

Get even more GABA

Food isn't the only way to produce more GABA; aerobic exercise also does the same job. It doesn't matter what the intensity is, just choose something that's doable for you. Research has shown that the beneficial effects on mood and sleep from yoga occur as a result of GABA activation.[32]

BODY
Understand Genitourinary Symptoms

Some of the conditions associated with perimenopause improve after the transition to the post-menopausal years. Unfortunately – and there's no gentle way to say this – genitourinary symptoms aren't one of them. This is a broad term that covers a variety of conditions in the pelvic region. For obvious baby-making reasons, there are more receptors for reproductive hormones here than anywhere else. This part of the body suffers more than any other as oestrogen, testosterone and progesterone decline.

It's important to remember that we're not just talking about painful sex here, but a whole range of symptoms that can make it uncomfortable even to wear jeans, or ride a bike or wear some types of underwear. Symptoms that have us rushing to the loo way more than we used to, or that result in accidents on the way. Symptoms that result in recurring infections or the tearing and splitting of vulval tissue. Horrendous issues that can, however, in many cases, be resolved.

Declining hormones, combined with ageing, result in a range of interrelated symptoms and conditions, defined as the Genitourinary Syndrome of Menopause (GSM). They may begin during perimenopause, or they may not appear until many years later – which is why people don't associate them with lack of oestrogen, and there's a tendency to suffer in silence. These are conditions that affect the vagina, vulva (i.e. everything we see on the outside of our genitals, such as the labia and clitoris) and urinary tract.

What we're talking about here are:

- Genital symptoms (dryness, burning, irritation and splitting)
- Sexual symptoms (lack of lubrication, discomfort or pain during sex)
- Urinary symptoms (frequency, urgency, incontinence, waking in the night to pass urine, pain, and recurrent urinary tract infections – UTIs)

Until relatively recently, the terms *vulvovaginal atrophy* and *atrophic vaginitis* were used to describe this set of symptoms. But in the last decade it has been recognised that they fail to fully describe the constellation of symptoms and signs associated with the genitourinary system after menopause, because they don't account for symptoms of the lower urinary tract.[33] It still astonishes me how long it's taken – and is still taking – the medical profession to catch up with women's health needs post-menopause. Getting the terminology right is a good start.

Statistics on how many women suffer genitourinary symptoms of menopause vary wildly – from 27 per cent of all women to a staggering 84 per cent.[34] Whatever the reality, it is likely to be underdiagnosed and undertreated – please don't let that be you. If any of these symptoms affect you, seek help. Dr Juliet Balfour told me, 'A lot of menopause symptoms do get better with time. However, the vaginal, vulval and urinary symptoms will only get worse and worse without treatment. Doctors aren't good at asking about this, and patients often don't mention these symptoms, but it is such an important thing to talk about.'

But don't panic: treatment can be straightforward – keep reading.

THE LINK BETWEEN GENITOURINARY ISSUES AND REPRODUCTIVE HORMONES

Women's health physio Christien Bird explained it to me like this: 'Our vaginal walls, and our bladder, have more oestrogen receptors than any other tissue in our bodies, so they're very, very reliant on oestrogen. When oestrogen declines, those muscles in the vagina and the pelvic floor are more impacted than any other tissue. The result is thinning of the labia, the bladder, the vaginal walls, and also a change in bladder function. On top of that, oestrogen changes the acidity level of the vagina. We have an acidic pH around our vagina and bladder entrance to fight off bacteria, but once we start losing oestrogen that pH becomes more alkaline. So we lose that protection, hence the increase in UTIs and other infections post-menopause.'

Research has shown that, post-menopause, several species of bacteria can invade the bladder walls, increasing the risk of UTIs.[35] UTIs account for 25 per cent of all infections in women, and after menopause the risk of an infection recurring rises to 55 per cent. Urinary tract infections (UTIs) are one of the most common infections in nursing homes.

HOW TO TREAT GENITOURINARY ISSUES

Christien explains, 'There are a few really nice studies now showing that the gold standard treatment is a combination of topical vaginal oestrogen and pelvic floor training. Both these treatments can also help with sexual experience.'

Pelvic floor training

She goes on, 'In terms of exercise, download the Squeezy app, which explains really clearly what to do. But if you're not sure, or it doesn't feel like it's working, go and see your GP and make sure you get referred to a women's health physio. It's hard to deal with pelvic floor problems by yourself if you have a serious issue, and I so want women to start asking for help.

'Women are such good "put-er up-ers"; they'll put up with painful sex, urinary and bowel incontinence, even prolapse. But there are no medals for putting up with things. No one's going to erect a statue because you've been so brilliant at putting up with symptoms all your life. So please, please go and talk to your GP or another healthcare professional.' Turn to page 94 for more on pelvic floor exercises.

Topical vaginal oestrogen

This is a form of hormone therapy, but is applied, usually via pessary or cream, directly to the vulva and/or vagina. It is now available in UK pharmacies, but it is not 'over-the-counter HRT', despite what some newspaper headlines have told us. Unlike the treatment we usually think of as HRT, vaginal oestrogen is not systemic and only affects the tissues it comes into close contact with. As Dr Balfour says, 'Topical vaginal oestrogen is a tiny dose, so small that a lot of women who've had breast cancer can have it.'

Dr Carys Sonnenberg adds, 'Topical vaginal oestrogen used inside the vagina can be used safely by almost everybody, whether they take HRT or not. It is important to understand the difference between oestrogen as part of Hormone Replacement Therapy, which is taken as a gel, patch, spray, oral tablet or implant, and topical vaginal oestrogen, which is placed into the vagina to help relieve vaginal, vulval and bladder symptoms, which are common in menopause.'

I've seen confusion about this in my own coaching groups. When one 65-year-old shared that a vaginal oestrogen prescription had sorted out her recurrent UTIs, another member of the group had an 'ah-ha' moment. She was suffering from vaginal and vulval soreness and dryness, but hadn't wanted to 'take HRT' when offered it by her doctor. Once she understood the difference between systemic and vaginal oestrogen, she was able to go back and have another conversation with her doctor and get the help she needed.

The joint position statement by the British Menopause Society, Royal College of Obstetricians and Gynaecologists and Society for Endocrinology on best practice recommendations for the care of women experiencing the menopause, *Post Reproductive Health*, published in October 2022, also backs the safety of vaginal oestrogen:

> *Low-dose and ultra-low dose vaginal oestrogen preparations can be taken by perimenopausal and menopausal women experiencing genitourinary symptoms and continued for as long as required. All vaginal oestrogen preparations have been shown to be effective in this context and there is no requirement to combine vaginal oestrogens with systemic progestogen treatment for endometrial protection, as low-dose and ultra-low dose vaginal oestrogen preparations do not result in significant systemic absorption or endometrial hyperplasia.*

Dr Balfour adds that we should be aware we need to keep taking vaginal oestrogen forever to continue to reap the benefits; it's not a finite course of treatment.

One other thing to bear in mind . . .

Although topical vaginal oestrogen doesn't work in the same way as systemic HRT – i.e. it only works in the tissues where it's applied, not the whole of our bodies – the leaflet that comes with it, in the packet, often gives the same warnings as we're given for systemic, oral oestrogen tablets.

Dr Balfour is very clear on the impact this can have. 'I have to warn women, particularly older women, who think "I don't want HRT" that the leaflet isn't accurate. I tell them they can read the leaflet if they want to, but not to panic because the warnings don't apply to local oestrogen. Otherwise, they go home, they read the leaflet, decide not to take it, and I've missed my chance to help them with their symptoms.'

OMEGA-7 supplementation

I don't want you to end up with a long list of supplements to consider once you've read this book – I'd always rather there were other lifestyle interventions you could consider first. However, there's some interesting research into the efficacy of omega-7 supplementation to reduce vaginal dryness. Omega-7 is an essential fatty acid, but not as well known as its siblings, omega-3 and omega-6. It's part of the natural structure of our skin and mucous membranes. The best external sources are oily fish like salmon and anchovies, macadamia nuts, avocados and a coastal shrub called sea buckthorn. Research has linked supplementation with 3g of sea buckthorn oil daily to a significant reduction in vaginal atrophy symptoms for post-menopausal women.[36] Another study, on the effect of a gel containing sea buckthorn oil, also found a reduction in vulvovaginal atrophy.[37]

BODY
Hot Flushes and Other Persistent Symptoms

If you are suffering persistent menopause symptoms, please, please talk to your doctor. If you're not happy with their response, or you feel you're not being listened to, ask to be referred to a specialist menopause clinic. There's no need to suffer in silence. Hormone replacement therapy (also known as menopause therapy) is the main medication available on prescription for menopause symptoms. It's suitable for many – but not all – women. Some women have medical histories that preclude the use of HRT, for others it doesn't work or causes side effects. This is a conversation for you and your doctor, but do make sure you're informed on the risks and benefits of HRT before your appointment.

Awareness of symptoms has changed dramatically in recent years, and you should now be able to get the help you need. All the protocols discussed in this book – good nutrition, regular movement, stress reduction and mindset – will also make a huge difference to your symptoms. And if you're on HRT, it will work more effectively if you have a healthy lifestyle.

HOT FLUSHES

When I surveyed followers of The Age-Well Project on their experiences post-menopause, one reported experiencing hot flushes 'for sixteen years and counting!' Another referred to them as 'useful in winter because I live in a cold house; not so good in summer'.

Hot flushes are just one of the many symptoms of menopause that may journey with us into the years beyond the final menstrual period. Oestrogen activates the hypothalamus, which controls body temperature. So what do we get when oestrogen declines? A body thermostat that's out of control. And, of course, as we traverse our power decade, we're getting older, so the effects of ageing combine with the symptoms of menopause.

Lifestyle options to reduce hot flushes

Aside from HRT, there are, of course, many other ways to tackle symptoms that persist post-menopause. HRT isn't the only answer, but it is the only one on prescription. There are plenty of lifestyle options to try, either on their own or to complement medication.

MEALS

Mediterranean diet

Research has shown that following the Mediterranean diet (see page 75) can help reduce hot flushes.[38] A high intake of fruit also helps.

Phytoestrogens

Soy: Soy is particularly high in isoflavones (plant-based phytoestrogens mainly found in beans), which bind to oestrogen receptors, mimicking our own oestrogen.

Black cohosh: This is a herb native to North America, which can be bought as a supplement. Small studies[39] of post-menopausal women have shown it to be effective for hot flushes. Research that compared its effectiveness with that of evening primrose oil found that both herbs reduced the severity of hot flushes, but black cohosh also reduced the number of incidents.[40]

Please note: Some phytoestrogen supplements may be linked to increased risk of breast cancer and other health issues for some women. Please talk to your doctor about any concerns you may have.

Find your food triggers

A hot flush can be triggered by a spicy meal, foods high in sugar and fat, caffeine and alcohol. Try keeping a food diary if you think this might apply to you, so you can work out which foods or drinks make the problem worse.

MOVEMENT

Mind-body connection

Stress exacerbates hot flushes, so anything that reduces stress, like yoga, meditation or mindfulness will help. Have a look at the stress section on page 149.

Keep your cool

If you can control the thermostat in your home or place of work, try to keep the temperature on the cool side. Dress in layers of natural fabric. Fay Reid, who I interview on page 42, curates a selection of good-looking clothes that work for this on her website, fayreid.com.

NIGHT SWEATS

Night sweats, part of the same vasomotor response to menopause that triggers hot flushes, are a great sleep disruptor for many women. Around 75 per cent of women experience these symptoms during the menopause transition and beyond. Try some of the lifestyle interventions listed above, as well as:

Keep bedding light . . .

Heavy duvets and blankets can trigger night sweats. If your sleeping partner complains about being cold, follow the lead of a GP friend of mine, who bought two single duvets for her double bed: a lightweight one for herself and a warmer one for her other half.

. . . And the bedroom cool

Turn down the thermostat at night, keep a fan by the bed, try a cool pad or pillow.

And one more thing . . .

Once we're post-menopausal (i.e. it's been a year since our final period), any vaginal bleeding is irregular bleeding. You need to talk to your doctor about this. There can be several causes of post-menopausal vaginal bleeding, and you want to be sure that it's one of those and not a symptom of uterine or ovarian cancer.

Post-menopausal bleeding can be caused by:[41]

- inflammation and thinning of the vaginal lining or womb lining, as a result of lower oestrogen levels
- cervical or womb polyps – growths that are usually non-cancerous

- a thickened womb lining (endometrial hyperplasia) – this can be caused by HRT, high levels of oestrogen or being overweight, and can be a precursor to uterine cancer

Treatment is available for all these issues, so please do get to your doctor as soon as you can.

BODY
Aches and Pains
Post-Menopause

Aching joints is one of the more surprising, and really not fun, symptoms of menopause. And it can persist into the post-menopause years too. As with so many health issues in our fifties and sixties, declining oestrogen plays a role. We have oestrogen receptors in the connective tissue of our joints, so when that protective cloak of hormones is removed, they're likely to stiffen. Oestrogen itself is anti-inflammatory. Add to this increasing inflammation throughout the body from general wear and tear, and the impact of ageing, and we've got a lot of aches to deal with.

Dr Carys Sonnenberg explains, 'As oestrogen levels fall, joints can become inflamed and painful, and symptoms from pre-existing arthritis may become worse. The neck, shoulders, elbows, hands, spine and knees are commonly affected in menopause. Osteoarthritis affects the structure of the joint; the cartilage thins and becomes rougher so the joint doesn't move as smoothly as it should. The main symptoms are pain and sometimes stiffness of the affected joints.'

There are, of course, other forms of arthritis: the term inflammatory arthritis is used as an umbrella term for axial spondyloarthritis and rheumatoid, psoriatic and reactive arthritis. All of these are autoimmune diseases, meaning the immune system attacks the cells lining our joints, making them stiff and painful. Dr Sonnenberg adds, 'If you're suffering with aches and pains in your joints, it would be sensible to get a check over from a doctor. I think the difficulty is that women put a lot of symptoms down to menopause. We must remember that two things can go on at the same time, so joint pain doesn't just have to be a menopausal symptom. There are also other things that can naturally go wrong with us at this time in our lives. It's important that women are given the message that, if you're in pain, and you've done everything you can, you must get a check over. You can't assume everything is due to menopause.'

Reducing stress (see page 149) and gentle stretching exercises, like yoga and tai chi, can help relieve mild aches and pains, as can regular walking. The critical point here is that we don't let low-level aches and pains stop us from moving regularly. No one wants to exercise through extreme pain, of course, but the less we move, the more likely we are to ache. And not moving is one of the worst things we can do for our post-menopausal health.

BODY
Eyes and Ears

EYES

Oestrogen is abundant in the human eye, so it's no surprise that declining levels impact both vision and eye health. There are oestrogen receptors in our tear glands, and tear production declines after menopause. Older women are more likely than older men to suffer dry eye syndrome. Several studies have, however, shown that dry eye improves with HRT.[42]

Dr Fionnuala Barton points out that dry eye is a condition that's really common as we get older, irrespective of the oestrogen perspective. She feels it's rather underplayed by the medical community, but can be enormously debilitating. It is treatable, though. She explains: 'Using eye drops consistently can completely revolutionise your experience. But you do need to be consistent. They need to be dropped in, morning and evening, every single day, in order to provide the appropriate kind of fat, rich lubrication across the eye that is then going to reduce the need for your eyes to produce watery tears. We see a kind of paradox where people with watery eyes make their dry eye condition much worse, because tear water is not rich in the lipids you need to maintain moisture on the surface of the eye. That oily film across the eye gets disrupted as we age, and certainly with oestrogen deficiency.'

In addition, oestrogen may be a potential factor in diseases that affect the retina, such as glaucoma and age-related macular degeneration (AMD). The risk of both of these increase after menopause. Cataract risk has also been linked to menopause. It may be that increased oxidative stress caused by the decline in oestrogen impacts cataract growth.[43] It's worth knowing that cataracts have a direct effect on the brain, as they reduce visual stimulation and make the patient more isolated – both of which erode cognitive resilience. But after cataract surgery, dementia risk returns to normal.

I asked a neuro-opthalmologist for simple tips for improved eye health and they advised:

- Close your eyes for five minutes at the end of every hour of screen time. That's a lot – I've been trying, and while it's nice to have a break, it does feel like a long time!
- Use hydrating eye drops, see page 141, because screen work leads to more evaporation from the eye's surface. I use preservative-free ones.

- Don't overthink it. A healthy diet and exercise make a huge difference to eye health, so don't get caught up in the minutiae.

When it comes to nutrition, getting enough omega-3 fatty acids, vitamins A, B, C, E and K and other antioxidants helps keep vision healthy. A research review that looked at carotenoids (antioxidants that give vegetables their colour) and their impact on women's eye and brain health found that high intake of the nutrients lutein and zeaxanthin (from leafy greens and yellow vegetables like corn) is linked to lower risk of macular degeneration and cataracts.[44] Sea buckthorn supplementation (see page 132) has also been linked to reduced symptoms of dry eye.

EARS

Just like our eyes, our ears and auditory pathways have oestrogen receptors, which means that our hearing can be impacted at menopause. Some women experience tinnitus (ringing in the ears) during perimenopause, possibly as a result of declining oestrogen levels causing confused messages to be relayed back to the brain. Low oestrogen may also impact hearing by causing alterations in blood flow to the cochlea. One study found that lower levels of estradiol were linked to less sensitive hearing in post-menopausal women.[45] There may also be a link between lower bone density and hearing loss as the bones of the inner ear start to weaken.

However, midlife can also be a time when hearing starts to decline naturally regardless of menopause status. If you're concerned about hearing loss, ask your doctor for a referral to an audiologist. And be aware that midlife hearing loss is a risk factor for dementia.

BODY
Dental Health and
Dry Mouth

Dry mouth (xerostomia) is one of those symptoms that becomes more prevalent as we age and get further away from our menopause transition. However, it's also linked to decreased oestrogen levels, so it can start in perimenopause. A dry mouth is caused by reduced saliva production. Saliva helps protect the mouth and teeth from bacteria, making us more prone to gum disease and tooth decay when levels decline. It also stimulates our taste buds and is the first stage in the process of extracting nutrients from food, so both our taste and digestion can also be impacted when levels are reduced.

The enzyme amylase, which is the most prevalent enzyme in saliva, helps break down starch from the moment we consume it, making it easier to digest. But if we don't have enough saliva, we may be lacking in amylase, making starchy carbohydrates more difficult to absorb in the gut.

Staying hydrated, chewing gum, plus avoiding too much caffeine, alcohol and salty, spicy foods, can help keep saliva production at optimal levels. Stress and anxiety can be linked to dry mouth. See page 149 for how to manage stress.

With less saliva to protect our teeth and gums, we're also more likely to experience tooth decay and receding gums. This, in turn, can lead to periodontal (gum) disease, which can seriously impact dental health. Research has found a correlation between the progression of periodontal disease and Alzheimer's.[46]

Another important element of post-menopausal dental health is to remember that if bone loss is occurring elsewhere in the body, it will be happening in the skull and jaw too. That can also impact our teeth. Studies have shown that post-menopausal women have a greater risk of tooth loss. There's also a correlation between osteoporosis and gum disease:[47] loss of bone density in the jawbone can make it easier for bacteria to penetrate. Turn to the section on bone health on page 217 for more.

BODY
Skin and Hair

Dry, crepey skin and thinning, brittle hair – the impact of hormonal decline on our outward appearance can be profound. Oestrogen receptors aid the production of collagen and elastin, which keep our skin firm and hair strong. Once we're post-menopausal, research shows that skin becomes less elastic, the strata corneum (the skin barrier) thickens and there's less ceramide – needed for suppleness – in the top layers of skin.[48] The skin barrier becomes compromised, which may explain why we're more prone to dryness, breakouts and sensitivity. With less pliable skin, lines become more noticeable and we're likely to experience sagginess around the jaw line.

Collagen supplements are heavily marketed towards women in menopause and beyond. There's some research that indicates that they can reduce wrinkles and improve hydration. Collagen may also support bone density and hair health, but, of course, these supplements come at a cost.

Oestrogen also keeps hair in its growth phase, helping make it thicker and stronger. Many people report thinning hair in menopause and this can be linked to lower levels of another reproductive hormone, progesterone. An enzyme that can cause hair loss is inhibited by progesterone, so once that declines we're more likely to experience shedding.

These changes can have a profound psychological effect too: we may feel we are 'losing' ourselves as our appearance alters. We've been culturally conditioned to put a value on how we look, and change can be hard to navigate. This is something make-up artist and psychotherapist Lee Pycroft finds with many of her post-menopausal clients: 'People become critical of themselves. When they look in the mirror, they may no longer identify with their reflection and struggle to accept the change in their appearance. The person they see on the outside doesn't reflect how they feel on the inside.' This leads to another question: are we wrong to care? 'People worry they're being superficial by caring about their appearance,' says Lee. 'But appearance is a reflection of other things going on in our lives. We need to think about how we show up in the world and believe, no matter how our appearance shifts, that our value as a person remains.'

There's no magic formula to repair post-menopausal skin and hair (imagine the profits if there was!), but experimenting with what works for us, moisturising EVERYTHING liberally and plenty of sunscreen can all help.

MIND
Do This First . . . Sort Out
Stress

Very few women get through the menopause transition without feeling stress or anxiety at some point. And the years that follow may be the same: research from India found that one quarter of post-menopausal women had high, or very high, levels of stress.[49] The transition itself is stressful, then add in the many complexities of midlife: growing families, career pressures, ageing parents, financial concerns . . . and we end up with a pretty toxic mix. That feeling of being overwhelmed, or unable to cope with mental or emotional pressure, becomes all too familiar.

Stress and anxiety are two different things. Stress is a reaction to a difficult situation that is actually happening; it's how you respond to a direct threat. Anxiety is a feeling of apprehension or dread in situations where there is no actual real threat and can be disproportionate to the situation faced. Unlike stress, anxiety persists even after a concern has passed. Neither of them feel great, of course.

Why do we have these unpleasant responses? It's actually our brain trying very hard to keep us safe from what it perceives to be a threat. Sudden or ongoing stress activates our nervous system, flooding the bloodstream with adrenaline and cortisol. These two stress hormones work to raise blood pressure, increase heart rate and spike blood sugar. These changes pitch our bodies into a 'fight or flight' response. This is super-useful if we want to outrun a sabretooth tiger, less useful in a traffic jam. Much of the stress we feel today is an age-old adaption to forms of danger we're no longer threatened by. The end result is that we're pitched into a state of chronic, long-term stress – responding to a bad day at work as if our lives were at risk.

THE LINK BETWEEN STRESS AND REPRODUCTIVE HORMONES

The emotional changes of menopause are as important as the physical ones. We know that oestrogen and progesterone work in harmony to keep us energised and happy during our reproductive years. Oestrogen is highly active in the parts of the brain linked to emotion, while progesterone buffers stress. Testosterone also lowers anxiety and functions as an antidepressant. When levels decline, so too does our mood.

Our adrenal glands are designed to produce some oestrogen to support our health post-menopause, but if we're stressed, they're too busy pumping out cortisol to make much-needed oestrogen. So, in effect, the body's back-up system for oestrogen fails just when we need it most. It's yet another reason to focus on stress reduction.

OTHER CAUSES OF STRESS IN THE POWER DECADE

We're not being chased by a sabre-tooth tiger, so why do we feel stressed? Why do we have the same response to things that won't physically kill us – like worrying about our children, our partners, our health or our work?

The simple answer is because we care! And that's a good thing. Take a moment to let that sink in: we're stressed because we care about something.

We may want to reframe stress in that context – it allows us to achieve things, to help, to care for people. It's our brains saying, 'This needs to get done.' I coach a course on stress and the stories of three attendees encapsulate this idea of stressing because we care. All three women were in their early sixties, and all had very different reasons for stress. One had a stressful job and was managing a difficult younger colleague; one was caring for her husband, who was unwell and struggling to adjust to the limitations brought on by his condition; and the third was making a long journey each week to visit her dementia-struck mum in a care home many miles away. The common thread here is that they all cared A LOT about the situation which caused their stress.

OUR STRESS 'SIGNATURE'

Psychologists talk about 'stress containers': we all have one, and they're all different sizes. Stress flows into the container and, the more stressed we are, the faster it fills up. When stress levels build up, the container overflows and we feel like we're drowning in stress. We all have a different response to that: what psychologists call our stress signature. I'm sure you know your own – it might be teariness, irritability, tiredness, or turning to caffeine or alcohol. These responses don't help empty the stress container; they instead block the flow of stress out of the container and make things worse.

POWER UP: SMALL DAILY HABITS TO SORT OUT STRESS

MINDSET

Bring awareness to stress

I talked to psychologist Dr Lucy Ryan, who suggests the first step towards managing stress is to bring awareness to it. She told me, 'Notice your triggers; work out what triggers an unhelpful state, and what you do when you're in that state. It's all about knowing how you navigate around that awareness.' She talks about a quadrant of stress, which has 'survive' and 'thrive' on one axis, with 'burn out' and 'recharge' on the other. 'Ask yourself how you can move around those and navigate to more positive, helpful places,' she adds. It's not always easy to do this by ourselves, but it starts with self-awareness and understanding that what we're experiencing is stress.

Changing our response to stress

When stress barrels headlong towards us, it's hard not to feel completely overwhelmed. We believe we have no control over our response to stress, often thinking, 'I feel like this because of stressful situation *X*'. Whereas, in fact, we feel like this because of our RESPONSE to stressful situation X. Does the difference make sense to you? We may not be able to change the source of our stress, but we can change our response. The first step is to understand that the stressor, and our feelings of stress, are not one and the same. We can evaluate our stress response with that in mind. Taking time for self-reflection, and asking ourselves sometimes difficult questions, helps us unpick and manage these feelings.

Caring for ourselves

To quote Audre Lorde, 'Caring for myself is not self-indulgence; it's self-preservation'. It isn't about spending money to solve your problems – it's about getting to the root of your issues and healing yourself. Dr Ryan puts it like this: 'It starts with some care and compassion for oneself, one's body, one's time. We need to work out how we want to be through our fifties and sixties, and find what will nurture us rather than dancing to everyone else's tune.'

Sustainable nurturing

Sustainable nurturing is about committing to look after ourselves as an act of self-respect. It requires regular check-ins, taking time for self-reflection and prioritising our own needs. Making sure we find a tribe of supportive people, getting outside, carving out time for hobbies and interests, developing a stress-reduction practice like meditation or yoga and prioritising sleep will all help us nurture ourselves. We need to build deliberate actions into our routines to make sure these things happen, as they won't occur by themselves.

Write an accomplishments list

We spend so much time fretting over what we haven't done, that we often don't stop to appreciate all we have accomplished in a day. It might be something that seems insignificant – like a dog walk or preparing a family meal – but they're all accomplishments that we can celebrate.

What do you need at work?

To navigate stress, we need to make positive choices for our physical, mental and emotional state. And that may include taking a long, hard look at our place of work. Dr Ryan works with a lot of corporations trying to hold on to older female workers. 'It's not as if many women can leave their place of work,' she says. 'They may be the breadwinner, raising teenagers, paying care fees for elderly parents. But some do, and they navigate a new life for themselves out of the corporate environment, setting up their own businesses when they see they're not given the flexibility they need in the workplace.'

How will you actively relax today?

Active relaxation is a powerful tool when we're seeking calm in our lives. It doesn't mean bingeing on TV or 'chilling'. It means meditation, breath work, walking, spending time with our community, gardening, colouring, journalling or crafts. Dr Ryan adds, 'Whatever it is you love, do more of it. Work out what turns you on – it could be writing, journalling, poetry, sculpture. Is there something you've wanted to do all your life and you've just never done it? Rather than thinking, "I should be doing yoga", work out what speaks to you. What do you want to put into your life that you've left out? That will help.'

Create a low-stress morning routine

Anchoring the day with a morning routine helps reduce stress. Try some of the ideas below to power up your day:

- No phone or social media for at least half an hour after you wake
- Make the bed
- Drink a glass of water
- Experience a moment of gratitude

- Move!
- Eat a healthy breakfast
- Get some daylight – my favourite start to the day
- Listen to some uplifting music or a podcast
- Hug someone or something – even yourself

MEALS

Understand the stress response

Stress triggers a series of biological responses in our bodies, including the release of stress hormones, an increase in blood sugar and a rise in blood pressure. The foods we eat have a huge impact on that stress response by steadying blood sugar levels, boosting resilience and supporting brain health.

Put calm on the menu

When our gut microbiota ferment fibrous foods, they make short-chain fatty acids, which are extremely powerful within the body. One of these fatty acids – butyrate – has been shown to be anti-inflammatory: it improves memory and mood, and reduces stress. Help your gut make butyrate by eating beans, oats, cold potatoes, apples, onions and leeks.

In addition, try some of these other stress-busting ingredients:

- Avocados are a great source of B vitamins, which we need for a healthy nervous system.
- Almonds contain vitamins B2 and E, which help boost the immune system in times of stress.
- Dark chocolate (70 per cent cocoa solids or above) is believed to help reduce stress (and it tastes good!).

Vitamin C

Studies suggest this vitamin can curb levels of stress hormones while strengthening the immune system. In one study, blood pressure, and elevated levels of the stress hormone cortisol, returned to normal more quickly when participants took vitamin C before a stressful task.[50] Make sure you're getting vitamin C from oranges, kiwi fruit and peppers.

Magnesium

This mineral helps reduce stress and increase relaxation. One cup of spinach helps you stock up on magnesium. Don't like spinach? Other green and leafy vegetables are also good magnesium sources. Try soy beans or a fillet of salmon, which are also high in magnesium. Transdermal magnesium flakes make for a relaxing bath-time soak.

Oily fish

To keep stress in check, make friends with naturally fatty fish. Omega-3 fatty acids, found in fish such as salmon and sardines, can prevent surges in stress hormones. For a healthy supply of feelgood omega-3s, aim to eat at least 100g of fatty fish at least twice a week.

Black tea

Drinking black tea may help us recover from stressful events more quickly. One study compared people who drank four cups of tea daily for six weeks with people who drank another hot drink.[51] The tea drinkers reported feeling calmer and had lower levels of the stress hormone cortisol after stressful situations. Unsurprisingly, this was a British study – I think any Brit could tell you that a cuppa is stress-relieving!

MOVEMENT

Box breathing

This is my favourite breathing exercise; I do it before every coaching session and live event. It's so simple and so calming. Just breathe in for a count of four, hold for a count of four, breathe out for four, then hold (with empty lungs) for four. And repeat. Imagine you're drawing a box as you're doing it – or draw a box with your finger as you go. Try to do it four times to calm and focus yourself.

Tone the vagus nerve

If there is a single key to health and happiness, it may be the vagus nerve. This nerve, or more accurately, bunch of nerves, connects most of the major organs between the brain and the colon and moderates our fight-or-flight response. It's largely responsible for the brain-body connection, and stimulating it (also known as toning) is the single best thing we can do to reduce stress and age-related inflammation. These actions stimulate the vagus nerve – try one, or all, of them:

- Deep, rhythmic breathing, like the box breathing exercise above.
- Laughing has a similar effect. What makes you laugh?
- Cold showers. Take it slowly, but cold showers are hugely beneficial for mind and body.
- Humming. The vagus nerve is connected to the vocal cords, so humming a tune, or a low 'om', stimulates it.

Mind-body movement

Movement where mind and body are in harmony, like yoga, tai chi and qi gong, is particularly beneficial when it comes to stress reduction. Studies have also shown that yoga can help with the management of menopausal symptoms.[52]

Find a form of movement that brings you joy

Exercise, in all its forms, reduces stress. If you begin with the mindset that it's beneficial and it's going to be fun, it will be. Find joy in movement, whether that's dancing round the kitchen, going for a long walk with a friend (rather than meeting up for a drink) or having a go with a skipping rope.

MIND
Anxiety and Other Persistent Symptoms

For many women, the psychological symptoms of menopause can be the hardest to cope with. That rollercoaster of emotion, from anger to tears and back again in a few minutes, is one of the most confusing and frustrating aspects of the menopause transition, and may last well beyond it.

We have to remember that symptoms of menopause begin in the brain, not in the ovaries. Just as each part of our bodies is changing, so too is our brain, and that has a knock-on effect on our mood and mental health. Oestrogen works as a messenger between our ovaries and brains, so, when levels drop, brain function can be impacted, leading to a decline in mental health. That 'fight or flight' response I talked about in the stress section is hardwired into the part of the brain called the amygdala. Oestrogen fluctuations here can cause low mood and anxiety.

ANXIETY, MOOD AND EMOTION

Oestrogen is also part of the process that creates serotonin, the feelgood hormone, in the brain. So low oestrogen means low serotonin, which means we need to work harder to support our own mental health. But, as Dr Fionnuala Barton points out, that's not all that's at play here. 'I think it's overly simplistic to say that it's all related to sex hormones. They're fluctuating and becoming deficient at a time in our lives when we're probably under quite a lot of stress. Most of us will be doing multiple things in our lives. And it's a sharp scorpion sting in the tail for hormones to decline at a time when we're often most in need of stability.'

She continues: 'The simple version is that we've got a wealth of oestrogen and testosterone receptors in important parts of the brain that are responsible for perception of fear. So we can become more susceptible to things that we see as a threat, but that we haven't been fearful of before, because our brain chemistry is changing and our nervous system isn't working in the way that it used to.'

The end result is that we perceive threats when there aren't any, and we can't regulate our emotions in the way that we used to. Hence the rapid change in emotions we sometimes experience. Dr Barton goes on, 'And then you've got other changes in the prefrontal cortex, for example, where our executive functions impact forward planning and decision making. And if your amygdala and hippocampus aren't necessarily firing well, you end up in this vicious circle of not being able to regulate emotion, which has an impact on outcome, and those outcomes having an impact on what you see as a threat.'

HRT can support the hormonal element of these issues, but we still need to look at how we modify our responses to the stresses we face post-menopause. See below for medical interventions and read the section on stress (page 149) for practical tips to try at home.

COGNITIVE BEHAVIOURAL THERAPY

Cognitive behavioural therapy, or CBT, is a practical form of psychotherapy focused on bringing awareness to the present moment and dissecting problems so we can change negative thought patterns. Working with a therapist, a CBT patient will break down problems into separate areas, and analyse responses to stressful situations. They then work together to change negative responses and apply these changes to everyday life. The number of sessions is finite – usually four or six – unlike 'regular' therapy, which is open-ended. It's been found to help with the vasomotor symptoms of menopause, as well as stress, low mood and insomnia. CBT can help us have calmer responses, or accept a situation we may be facing.

THE ROLE OF ANTIDEPRESSANTS

In recent years, there have been many reports of women being offered antidepressants by doctors who fail to diagnose perimenopausal symptoms. Dr Barton believes that, 'Despite them being a useful part of a holistic strategy to improve mental health symptoms in perimenopause and menopause, there remains substantial stigma around the use of these medications in this context in comparison with the widespread reduction in stigma associated with these drugs for treatment of primary mental health issues, which often coexist or predate perimenopause. They can be a useful part of the armoury or toolkit and can be life-saving in cases where women experience suicidal thoughts, which is sadly common. Like HRT, though, antidepressants are not without side effects, so it is important their use is carefully considered in collaboration between patients and their clinicians.'

MIND
Low Libido

This was another issue mentioned by many women in my survey of Age-Well Project followers. For obvious reasons, it can have a devastating effect on our sense of self and our relationships. Some of the causes of low libido in our fifties and sixties relate to the increased risk of genitourinary problems (see page 125 for more on this), but they're not the only issue.

Dr Juliet Balfour told me, 'There are so many different factors that impact libido. Certainly, if genitourinary symptoms have caused dryness and soreness, so it's going to hurt when you have sex, obviously that's going to affect your libido. But then you've got so many other things. You've got your hormone levels, your relationship, how tired you are, how stressed you are, whether you've had previous difficult experiences, what you feel about your body image – all that goes into libido.'

Hormone therapy can help with this. She goes on: 'Certainly, hormones can have an effect. By far the most important thing is to get the oestrogen levels right with a suitable dose of transdermal oestrogen. And then, obviously, there's a lot of talk about testosterone. This can be controversial, but, understandably, a lot of women want to try it to see if it is the missing link for them. If the current HRT is optimised and there are no other obvious issues in the relationship or the other things I've mentioned, a trial of testosterone can be a good idea.

'For some women, it makes a big difference, for others it doesn't make any difference at all. We particularly need to offer testosterone to younger women who have had their ovaries removed, as they're the ones that may benefit the most from this. We need more research to assess the other possible benefits of testosterone supplementation.'

INTIMACY

Intimacy is about the connection between two people; it's not (necessarily) about sex. The hormonal changes of menopause can result in low libido, and it may also have affected our feelings of intimacy with others. Creating intimacy is about trust and a feeling of safety – when two people support each other with affection and love. We need to make time to connect to loved ones: supporting each other through change and showing physical affection.

MIND
Brain Fog

Menopause has a dramatic effect on energy metabolism in the brain, which in turn can have a dramatic impact on how we perceive our brain is working. I want to make it super-clear right here that the brain fog that can come with the menopause transition is NOT an indication of early onset dementia (whatever it might feel like). Many of the brain-related symptoms that we experience during menopause do ease. Dr Juliet Balfour says, 'We do know that brain fog doesn't go on for ever and our brains do recalibrate and it goes away.' And many women report feeling greater mental clarity, and having better cognition, as they move through their fifties.

SIX TIPS FOR POST-MENOPAUSAL BRAIN FOG

1. Prioritise sleep – do everything you can to optimise sleep quality, going to bed and getting up at regular times, keeping your bedroom cool and dark.

2. Find time to rest and unwind, walk in nature, practise meditation or mindfulness – anything that allows your brain to switch off and be in the moment.

3. Stimulate your brain with new ideas, places and people. Our brains love novelty and experiencing new things helps cut through that 'cotton wool' feeling of brain fog.

4. Try puzzles, sudoku, crosswords, Wordle – anything that engages your brain and keeps it working. Don't do the same thing every day – mix it up to keep challenging yourself.

5. Feed your brain omega-3-rich foods, like oily fish, walnuts and flax seeds.

6. Try a Lion's Mane supplement. This Chinese mushroom has been linked to better cognition.

There's more on taking care of our brains on page 227.

MIND
Owning Our Age

The biggest gift we can give ourselves at this point in our lives is acceptance. Accepting that change will happen, finding time to reflect on it, reframing our negative thinking and staying in the moment will all help. We're ageing in an ageist world: I talk to so many women who fear they're invisible, that being in their fifties and beyond means they're no longer relevant. It's difficult to own our age when society conditions us that to be young is to be strong, desirable and beautiful. But the power decade is all about reclaiming that narrative and feeling the best we can.

I talked to podcaster and campaigner Karen Arthur about this. She suffered anxiety and depression through her menopause. I asked her what she would say to a woman who was struggling to own her age in her fifties or sixties. She told me, 'I would always say "get silent"; ask yourself what you really want and ask yourself your motives for doing things. I would say, write that stuff down. Journalling every morning for me is about getting all the anxiety out, getting it on paper. The thing about morning pages is that it's the third page where the truth comes out! Ask yourself how you're really feeling. But that needs a certain amount of silence. You have to choose yourself: you have to say, "I'm worthy of this time." I started to not hold on to society's expectations of getting older. My answer is always going to be, "get silent", because when you get silent you can allow yourself to really think about what you want.'

She continues: 'We don't know how powerful we are because we've had it socialised out of us. Women are incredible! But patriarchy, white body supremacy, capitalism, fear – which keeps us going back to the shops and buying things we don't need – all these things keep us small. Society's fixation with youth will kill us. So, for me, to be ageing like this – I'm proud. I feel that as older women we have almost a duty, a calling, to make sure we live the best life we can live, so that our kids, and their mates and all the women coming up across a diverse range of demographics recognise they can give themselves permission to do so too.'

You can read more from Karen on page 174.

Power Women: Kanan Thakerar

Kanan, 59, is a wonderfully gifted Yoga Nidra teacher. Nidra is a form of guided meditation known as yogic sleep. It's a beautiful, deeply calming practice where participants relax while the teacher guides them using imagery and affirmations to create a positive state of consciousness. Kanan discovered Nidra after a midlife health crisis left her too fatigued even to walk, forcing her to take early retirement from a job she loved.

Kanan was working as a purser for a major airline when she was taken ill. 'My body just started to pack up. I saw many, many doctors and initially they thought it was cancer, the next week it was Crohn's disease, the next week something else – each week they were coming up with something different. The only people I saw were doctors, because physically I was so weak I couldn't go anywhere. I had to move in with my mum because I couldn't look after myself; she had to look after me. I'd go for a shower and collapse, I was so badly fatigued. Then the last doctor said he'd tried everything, but he thought it could be lupus. He gave me twenty-six blood tests. One came back borderline, so he wanted to repeat them all. At that point I said, "Stop, I don't want any of this. I just need to stop." It had been seven months of doctors and tests. I decided to start doing ten minutes of yoga, just ten minutes. I would sit and stretch.'

Kanan travelled to New York for further treatment. 'While I was there I decided I needed community, so I joined a yoga centre near where I lived. The only yoga I could do was the gentle restorative type, and even that I found difficult. That's when I discovered Yoga Nidra. I started by doing one or two sessions, then three or four a week. And within eight weeks I was walking twenty blocks. I'd lost a stone in weight. My head was clearer. I was happier, I had less brain fog, my cognition was better. In every Yoga Nidra session I set the same intention: "I am healthy." It never changed. I just stuck with "I am healthy", because without your health, you don't have your job, and without your job, you don't have your home. Health is the central piece. When my health went, everything went.

'I was determined to get better. I wasn't going to stay where I was because I love life, I love people, I love experiences, I love travel. I just had to surrender and give myself time to heal. I was pensioned out of my job, so I used my pension to buy rental property. This meant I could support myself and have the time to heal. When my choice was sink or swim, I decided to swim.'

Kanan trained as a Yoga Nidra teacher herself and now runs classes. 'I feel very grateful for my life now. Really, truly grateful. It's like a second life, another chance. What I do now is so far away from what I did before. I love having the freedom to run my own show.'

I asked Kanan what she would say to women who want to make a big shift in their lives in their fifties, as she did. She told me, 'Just trust, really. This is not a dress rehearsal, so don't be scared – because every time you make a mistake, or something doesn't work out, there's always a reason. Whatever floats your boat, give it a shot, you've got nothing to lose.'

Yoga Nidra is a wonderful practice to support health post-menopause both physically and mentally. 'It's a complete game changer,' says Kanan. 'We don't take time for ourselves, that's the biggest thing. Nidra allows you an hour or two for yourself each week. It's activating the parasympathetic nervous system and each hour gives you the equivalent of four hours' sleep, four hours of restorative sleep nourishment. It releases stress, it releases tension, it just restores you. It's as if we are vessels, and when the vessel gets full, we need to release. And when you do Nidra, the release comes. It allows the body to process and heal on a very deep level, and your energy to connect. And it's so simple, you just have to lie down and allow your body to rest and restore. And that is so, so powerful. It makes you very much more creative. You have much more focus and it brings you into flow as the observer rather than as the reactor.

'I love what I do, I love what I have. I'm truly grateful for this chance.'

Find Kanan at www.kananyogabliss.com and @kananyogabliss on Instagram and Facebook.

Power Women: Karen Arthur

When I started thinking about the essence of the power decade, it was women like Karen, 60, I had at the front of my mind. She's used her experience of breakdown during menopause to recalibrate her life, giving up her career as a teacher after nearly thirty years and building a life that gives her joy: founding the Wear Your Happy movement, launching the podcast *Menopause Whilst Black*, sewing, campaigning and public speaking. When I spoke to Karen, she'd just made a major post-menopausal pivot by selling up in London and following a long-held dream to move to the sea.

I start by asking Karen why she'd made this major move. 'I could have been very comfortable in my house in London and stayed there for ever,' she replies, 'but I wanted to shake things up a bit. I feel that if you get too comfortable, it's time to do something else. I'm excited and I have no idea what's happening next. I feel open, and I've never been more sure – I've made some good decisions in my life and this is definitely up there. But I'm also in the habit of never regretting things, because all the things that happen, all the ups and downs and in between, make us the people we are.

'My own wisdom comes from age; it comes from anxiety and depression; it comes from a breakdown, which is also a break-through; it comes from leaving teaching. It comes from having the time and the space to think and be silent and get quiet for the first time ever. I was fifty-two when I finally left – or had to leave – my teaching job. I was signed off sick because I'd had a fall and wasn't being supported. No one was talking about menopause. I went to the doctor because the whole of my side was seizing up; I was limping and later on had to walk with a stick. I talked about my anxiety and depression and then I said I'm having hot flushes, I haven't had a period for a year, I think I'm menopausal. She offered me antidepressants.

'I decided to try other things before I would accept the anti-depressants. For the first time, I put myself first. I learned to say no, I learned to meditate, I went into therapy. That was a big deal, because I spent years knowing I should go, but thinking it was too expensive. Therapy should be free for all people. And I found this incredible Black woman and I didn't realise at the time how important that would become. Now I advocate for anyone, particularly people of colour, to find a therapist who looks like you, who you don't have to explain yourself to. I deepened my yoga and stretching practice. I decided to wear the clothes that make me happy, which evolved into the Wear Your Happy movement.

'I made a conscious decision to build my life up again in the way that I wanted, and I started with the affirmation that I would be very much kinder to myself. I don't bad-talk myself at all. I always say: ask yourself what you really want. Society tells us that menopausal women have no use: the subliminal message is "go quietly". I just know I'm not having that – it's why I stopped dying my hair, it's why I wear what I want, it's why I moved. If I'm here for one time, I can honestly say, if I was run over tomorrow, I'm living the best life. I want women to recognise that they can create the life they want by dreaming huge. Ageing is hard, but when we let go of expectations, it's like a snake, shedding.'

Karen started her podcast, *Menopause Whilst Black*, in 2020. 'George Floyd put a fire under me. *Menopause Whilst Black* is me finding my voice and owning my journey as a Black woman. And I was thinking about how menopause can be brought on by stress. And racism is stress. I wondered how Black women were coping with this, seeing husbands, brothers, uncles, people who look like us, being murdered. It's called racial weathering, which is the physical and mental effect of racism, of living in a White body supremacist world, seeing racism, seeing people being mistreated, mishandled, killed. I wanted to share Black British women's experiences. That's how it started, and no podcast had had two older Black women talking about menopause ever before in the UK.

'My priority now, at sixty, is always my mental wellbeing and my physical wellbeing. Life is out there; ageing is a privilege. Go out there and grab it by whatever you grab it by, set your boundaries, get silent, do what works for you and the people who matter. When we live the way we're meant to, when we show up, we empower all the people coming up behind us.'

Find Karen at www.thekarenarthur.com and @thekarenarthur and @menopausewhilstblack on Instagram.

SECTION 4

YOU HAVE THE POWER: REDUCE THE RISK OF LONG-TERM HEALTH ISSUES

Introduction

The menopause transition brings with it, for the vast majority of women, an array of all-too-obvious symptoms. But 'behind the scenes' there are a wide range of asymptomatic changes that will affect our health for the rest of our lives. The trajectory towards the chronic diseases of older age is faster and stronger in women for the simple reason that we have a pronounced drop-off in hormones in midlife. Once we are past our final menstrual period, we need to be laser-focused on reducing our risk of the chronic conditions of ageing, like weight gain and insulin resistance, diabetes, osteoporosis, arthritis, cardiovascular disease, dementia and cancer. It's a hefty list, but we can do much to reduce those risks, and that's what this section is all about.

Of course, we would ideally have been focused on reducing our risk regarding these chronic conditions for the last couple of decades. But it's difficult to focus on our long-term cardiovascular health, or dementia risk, when we're battling perimenopausal symptoms. We're more focused on not having a hot flush during an important meeting or managing fatigue while dealing with a young family. One of my clients said to me, 'I wish I'd started focusing more on my health ten years ago!' I reminded her that she's in her mid-fifties, with a pre-teen child. A decade ago, she was wrangling a toddler and coping with perimenopause. Not necessarily the time to be working on a long-term health strategy.

When oestrogen declines, we lose its protective power over our bones, hearts, brains and much more. Now it's up to us to look after ourselves. And if we're on HRT, we get back the hormones we've lost, but we don't get back the youth. As Dr Juliet Balfour explains, 'HRT replaces what the body needs oestrogen-wise, but it's still very important to look after our bodies as they age.'

In this section we look at some of the chronic, long-term conditions of ageing, how declining oestrogen – and other factors – impact our risk of getting them, and how we can power up, and feel the best we can. You'll notice lots of crossover – good sleep and stress reduction support pretty much every health condition, for example. The key, as always, is to work out what's doable for you, not let it become overwhelming and be kind to yourself.

Do This First . . . Understand Cardiometabolic Health

The unwieldly, and rather inelegant, phrase 'cardiometabolic health' describes a combination of factors that impact us at menopause. It refers to a double whammy of heart and blood vessel issues – hence the 'cardio' bit – and weight gain with increased diabetes risk, which is the 'metabolic' bit. The combination of the dramatic hormone shift women experience in midlife, plus the simple fact that we're getting older, means that this should be a key focus when we prioritise our long-term health.

The Lancet medical journal describes menopause as a 'cardiometabolic turning point for women'. Dr Fionnuala Barton explains, 'Perimenopause and menopause have a profound impact on our metabolic health. As we transition, we go through an enormous shift in metabolic health too, which we don't truly understand yet. There is a wealth of research indicating that sex-hormone changes precipitate changes in metabolic hormones and a substantial "metabolic shift" that in turn increases cardiovascular risk, diabetes risk and predisposition to weight gain.'

She adds, 'There is a very heavy focus on replacing oestrogen, because then we're reducing cardiovascular disease risk. But actually the priority should be achieving and maintaining good metabolic health in midlife. That might be a bigger part of the picture rather than purely focusing on the hormone deficiencies themselves.'

Dr Carys Sonnenberg is clear on the first steps we need to take to address this. 'It is important that women have a health check at midlife. This includes a fasting blood sugar, fasting lipids, blood pressure and height and weight. With this information we can look at risk factors and give advice and support to women with the necessary lifestyle changes needed to protect their metabolic and cardiovascular health.'

For simplicity, I've divided the broad subject of 'cardio-metabolic health' into two sections – weight gain and insulin resistance, and heart health.

Manage Weight Gain and Insulin Resistance

I've yet to meet a woman in her fifties or sixties who hasn't had a complex relationship with food at some point in her life. We're used to a narrative of diets, denial and punishment. In the power decade we need to create a more nurturing approach, where we're kind to our bodies, and where we support our health while adjusting to our changing hormones.

There can't be many people who head into the post-menopausal years without some awareness that their metabolism is changing. On average, we gain a pound and a half (700g) each year during our forties and fifties. In the USA, three-quarters of women are overweight or obese by the time they hit sixty. In the UK, we're not far behind, with over two thirds of women overweight or obese between the ages of fifty-five and sixty-four.[53]

The other major change is where that weight goes. Like many women, I've seen my fat stores – which happily sat on my hips until my forties – take up residence around my middle, post-menopause. That central body fat is made up of truncal fat and visceral fat. Visceral fat has the ability to wrap itself around our internal organs and cause profound health issues, particularly an increased risk of cardiovascular disease. Obese post-menopausal women have a higher chance of death from all causes and greater cancer risk.

Of course, not everyone puts on weight post-menopause. I've coached some tiny women who struggle to keep weight on and that's a very different issue. But for the majority of us, weight settles round our middle. This isn't a vanity issue; there are profound implications for our health. Dr Carys Sonnenberg explains, 'It is so important for women in midlife to have a look at their lifestyle choices, to protect their future health. Obesity comes with increased risk of Type 2 Diabetes, coronary heart disease, stroke and some types of cancer such as breast cancer and bowel cancer.'

Research published in autumn 2022 found key differences between inflammation and blood sugar control in women pre- and post-menopause.[54] Post-menopausal women also consumed more dietary sugars and reported worse sleep, both of which increase risk for type 2 diabetes, obesity and cardiovascular disease.

WHAT IS INSULIN RESISTANCE?

Weight gain and insulin resistance are, of course, two different things. But statistics show that almost half of obese women are also insulin resistant,[55] and the weight gain of midlife often triggers the condition. However, skinny people can be insulin resistant too. It's linked to the process that breaks carbohydrate down into glucose to use as energy. When glucose enters our bloodstream it triggers the release of insulin from the pancreas. Insulin also travels round the bloodstream, telling cells to take the glucose and make use of it. Once the glucose gets into our cells, it fuels our mitochondria, the cells' batteries, which fire up and use it as energy.

But if we consume more carbohydrate than our mitochondria need, they respond 'Thanks but no thanks' when insulin comes to call. This leads the pancreas to think that our cells aren't listening, so it churns out more insulin and our cells become increasingly resistant. Meanwhile, insulin is thinking, 'What am I going to do with all this spare energy?', and lays it down as fat stores instead. Which was great, when we were roaming the savannah and needed to store fat for winter, but not so useful these days.

Other factors have a role in our body's response to insulin too: a sedentary lifestyle, genetics, sleep disruption, inflammation and low levels of omega-3 fatty acids can all play a part. There's more on these later in this section and in the chapters on movement (page 83), sleep (page 111) and inflammation (page 243).

In particular, insulin resistance is the precursor to type 2 diabetes, and a component of cardiometabolic disorders,[56] that combination of heart issues and blood glucose problems explained in the previous section. People are three times more likely to be obese or have metabolic syndrome after menopause than before it.

However, get it clear in your mind that weight gain post-menopause is not all your fault: it's hardwired into our DNA as we age and as reproductive hormones decline. Dr Juliet Balfour explains, 'We lose our muscle mass when we lose our oestrogen; our basal metabolic rate goes down, so we're burning fewer calories when at rest. Plus, our body is desperate for oestrogen so it produces more abdominal fat because that produces a weak, and rather inflammatory, form of oestrogen. So it's our metabolism doing this to us.'

THE LINK BETWEEN WEIGHT GAIN, INSULIN RESISTANCE AND REPRODUCTIVE HORMONES

Pre-menopause, oestrogen helps take fat to our bums, hips and thighs. It takes precedence over other sex hormones, androgens, which promote the accumulation of abdominal fat. But as oestrogen declines, androgens get priority – resulting in fat that sits around our middles. Oestrogen also helps transport glucose to muscles, where it's used more effectively than if it's allowed to sit around in our bloodstream.

The form of oestrogen that we lose during menopause, estradiol, is the one that helps regulate metabolism and weight. There are receptors for estradiol in the hypothalamus region of the brain, which also controls appetite. The activity of ghrelin, the hunger hormone, seems to be reduced in the hypothalamus when oestrogen is present.[57] Meaning that, when oestrogen declines, our hunger cues are disrupted, and it's easier for us to overeat.

To add fuel to the fire, as it were, the form of oestrogen we can produce post-menopause, estrone, is made in fat cells. So it stands to reason that our bodies want to hang on to some fat to make sure that we are able to produce a bit of much-needed oestrogen, even in the weakened form of estrone.

Oestrogen and progesterone work together to help make the pancreas more sensitive – which is why our blood sugar response fluctuates through the menstrual cycle. Remember that pre-period sugar craving? That was progesterone acting on the pancreas. As these hormones decline, so does that sensitivity.

And, as always, we need to remember that insulin is a hormone, and all hormones work together throughout our bodies in a carefully choreographed routine. When one declines, others are thrown out of whack too.

OTHER CAUSES OF WEIGHT GAIN AND INSULIN RESISTANCE

Ageing

It's easy to lay all the blame for midlife weight gain on menopause. But ageing, in general, has a huge role to play. Both men and women gain weight in midlife, and women gain weight at roughly the same rate through their forties and fifties, regardless of menopausal status.

As we get older, we naturally lose lean muscle. On average, people can lose around 30 per cent of their muscle between the ages of fifty and seventy. Muscle burns more energy than fat, so it makes sense that we are more likely to have surplus calories as muscle declines.

Declining nutritional sensitivity

Our highly tuned digestive system is calibrated to 'read' our energy intake, managing it appropriately and making sure we have the energy we need, when we need it. But as we age, this system becomes less sensitive, leaving us prone to more fat storage.

Comfort eating

By the time we're post-menopausal, we have all kinds of emotional burdens and stressors to carry. We may have spent decades seeking comfort in food. When we eat sugar and highly fatty foods, our brain releases chemical rewards to help us feel better. We know that food doesn't cure our ills, but eating for comfort becomes a learned response and may be a way we've self-soothed since childhood. That's a very hard habit to break, particularly as we experience perimenopause. It becomes very easy to want something sweet with every meal, every cup of tea or coffee. The recommended daily intake of sugar is just six teaspoons a day.

Increased stress

As above, our stress response may be to reach for food. This may be a behaviour we've followed for decades. Plus, when we're stressed, our adrenal glands are so busy pumping out cortisol, the stress hormone, that they have little opportunity to make any oestrogen – something they're wired to do post-menopause. Instead, our bodies have to make oestrogen in belly fat. So the more stressed we are, the more our bodies hang on to that belly fat to make any oestrogen they can.

A University College London research paper found that people were more likely to become heavily overweight after a period of prolonged chronic stress.[58] They found that higher levels of the stress hormone, cortisol, correlated with increased weight and higher BMI. Cortisol also plays an important role in decisions about where fat is stored, taking it to that mid-section of the body.

Reduced physical activity

As we age, we become less physically active, meaning we burn less energy. A study looking at twins found that, of all the environmental factors affecting weight, physical activity is the most important.[59] Research into the activity levels of women aged fifty to sixty-four found that around half reported regular physical activity and only one quarter undertook strengthening exercises.[60]

And looking at women more broadly, a UK-based survey published in summer 2022 revealed that almost half of the female population had done no vigorous exercise in the previous year.[61] What's at the root of this? Covid, a lack of affordable childcare, a hangover from the days when we were told that sport wasn't for us, the awkwardness of exercise with others when we're out of shape? Or a combination of many factors?

Poor sleep

Research published in summer 2022 pointed to a vicious cycle for women aged forty to sixty-four, linking poor sleep, comfort eating and increased BMI.[62] All very familiar, all very understandable. When we're exhausted, we're much more likely to reach for a quick energy hit to keep us going, and less likely to want to exercise.

Societal pressures

We know that society doesn't value ageing women in the way it should. If we're undervalued, who's to blame us for reaching for a treat – something to make the world seem a slightly brighter place, albeit momentarily. Add to that the availability of hyper-palatable high-sugar and high-fat foods, marketed in such a way that it's 'just a treat'. No wonder we can't resist at the checkout.

A multibillion-pound industry has grown up around keeping our sweet tastebuds happy. By eating sugar we're buying into a false narrative that it's just a harmless treat – which it's not, if, ultimately, it makes us unhappy.

History of dieting

We may have been dieting on and off for decades by the time we reach our fifties. Diets give us an impossible framework to follow for the short term, and then make us feel terrible for not sticking to them. The very nature of dieting being a short-term activity sets us up for failure, because that's not what food is for. And diets disempower us from making choices about our food and what's best for us.

POWER UP: SMALL DAILY HABITS TO MANAGE WEIGHT GAIN AND INSULIN RESISTANCE

MINDSET

Examine how you think about your body

Diet and exercise may be the obvious things to think about when we consider weight gain, but how we think about our bodies in menopause is a critical component to this. Do we feel we deserve to look and feel our best? What's our mindset around our weight and what we eat?

Accept cravings

So often clients tell me that their good intentions around food are derailed by cravings. It's a catch-all term, designed to make us feel that we're at fault for wanting to eat certain foods, particularly sugary, processed foods. But as we've discussed on the previous page, the reality is very different. We're hardwired to seek sweet foods, and they're constantly pushed at us by a multibillion-pound industry that profits from exploiting our desires. We need to understand, first and foremost, that cravings aren't wrong. We need to start by accepting them. They're normal, not a failure!

You don't have to make cravings go away, but you also don't have to eat because of them. Think in terms of acceptance rather than suppression. There's no point trying to rely on willpower – that's just pushing the problem further down the track. Better to accept and examine those feelings. I encourage my clients to work through the process below:

- Give the craving a name. Tell yourself, 'I'm feeling that I want to eat/drink XX.'
- Allow yourself to feel the craving, don't ignore it.
- Sit with it. Give it ten minutes – how do you feel now?

Eat mindfully

Mindfulness is focusing on the present moment, while calmly acknowledging and accepting your feelings, thoughts and bodily sensations. Mindful eating is the process of paying attention to what we consume. It's so easy to grab food at our desk, in the car or on the run and barely pay it any attention. Bringing mindfulness to eating unravels that habit, inviting us to bring all our senses to any meal or snack.

I know it's easier said than done, but take the time to appreciate what you're eating. Put your plate in front of you and focus on it for a moment before you start eating. Ask yourself what you appreciate about it, how much you're looking forward to eating it and remind yourself of the health benefits (or not) without triggering guilt. Take a moment to feel gratitude for the food in front of you.

Then eat with intention, chewing properly and paying attention to every mouthful rather than swallowing mindlessly.

Find your joy

It's all too easy to become such a slave to our to-do list, job or just day-to-day life that the only time we allow ourselves a break is when we eat. Can you build other moments of joy and relaxation into your day? And in particularly stressful situations, eating may be the only self-soothing mechanism we can call on. What else can you try?

MEALS

Pay attention to what's in your food

Ultra-processed, ultra-palatable foods are designed to make us consume a lot and they have very little nutritional value. Research published in 2022 linked higher consumption of ultra-processed foods to more intense vasomotor symptoms and worse brain fog in post-menopausal women.[63] My clients find that when they start paying attention to what's actually in their meals, and understand the health benefits of whole, unprocessed foods, their shopping and eating habits change dramatically.

Healthy foods that are really easy to overeat

Just because a food is deemed healthy it doesn't mean we won't gain weight if we eat a lot of it. Watch out for the following foodstuffs – they're all delicious and packed with beneficial nutrients, but we shouldn't eat too much of them:

- Nut butters
- Dried fruit
- Avocado
- Aged cheese
- Dark chocolate

Keep hydrated

It's so easy for our bodies to confuse thirst for hunger, particularly as we get older and our thirst cues are less pronounced. Start the day with plenty of water – add a slice of lemon for a refreshing way to wake up.

Cinnamon

Cinnamon is a delicious spice loaded with health-promoting antioxidants. Studies suggest that consuming cinnamon may enhance insulin sensitivity and decrease insulin levels. It also brings sweetness to food without adding any sugar.

Swaps and swerves

What can you swap in to replace what you're craving? Herbal teas, kombuchas? Sweet potatoes instead of sweets? Try a liquorice tea after dinner – it's naturally sweet, so reduces the urge to grab a dessert. Green tea in the afternoon is also great, as it contains high amounts of an antioxidant known as epigallocatechin gallate (EGCG). Several studies suggest this may help fight insulin resistance.

Consume healthy fats

Essential fatty acids (EFAs) like omega-3s help balance insulin regulation. Find EFAs in oily fish like salmon and tuna, flax seeds and eggs – or take a marine algae supplement if you don't consume animal products.

Protein and fibre: every meal, every snack, every day

These two beauties, protein and fibre, help keep us feeling full and satiated. If we start the day with a sugary, low-fibre breakfast, we'll quickly find our blood sugar dipping and a craving for more carbs setting in. Start the day with protein and fibre – think eggs and wholewheat toast or Greek yogurt and oats – and blood sugar will be steady throughout the day.

MOVEMENT

Flip the script

Don't exercise to lose weight – we need to flip the script on that. Exercise should be for the joy of it, to make us strong and to build the muscle that will power us through our post-menopausal years. But there's no denying it: exercise burns energy. Muscle uses more energy than fat. And if we want to keep weight gain and insulin resistance under control, we need movement to be part of our lives.

Strength train

Muscle acts as a sponge to mop up glucose in the blood. One study found that post-menopausal women who underwent a twelve-week strength-training programme had reduced insulin levels and lower markers for cardiometabolic syndrome.[64] But don't throw yourself into a weights room without the right support and training – see the Movement chapter in Section 2 for more details.

Walk daily

There's really no end to the benefits of a daily walk. It can help move glucose to muscles, and it doesn't take a long hike to do it – ten minutes can bring huge benefits. In fact, it's actually better to break up the walks into smaller chunks – see below.

Move after meals

A 2022 review paper by the University of Limerick showed that movement after meals helps muscles absorb glucose, which keeps blood sugar levels stable.[65] Researchers analysed the results of seven studies that compared the effect of sitting, standing, or walking after eating. They found that – when it comes to glucose management – standing is better than sitting and walking is better than standing. Fifteen minutes was the perfect amount of time for a walk, but even two minutes made a difference.

HIIT

HIIT – high-intensity interval training – helps stimulate muscles to take up glucose from the blood to use as fuel, so blood sugar levels decrease. HIIT might sound, well, intense, but, in its simplest form, it's about increasing the intensity of the movement we do. So that could be walking faster for short bursts, or cycling harder, or doing short sets of exercise in the gym with rest periods in between.

Heart Your Heart

Of all vital organs impacted by the menopause transition, it's perhaps our hearts that are most affected. Oestrogen weaves its protective cloak particularly tightly around our tickers, so when it declines they're especially vulnerable.

Cardiovascular disease (CVD) is still the leading cause of death across the world,[66] and is now killing more people than ever before. Coronary heart disease (when the arteries that supply the heart muscle with blood become blocked) was the single biggest killer of women worldwide in 2019.[67] Rates of heart disease fatalities are increasing among women in midlife[68] and it now kills a larger proportion of women over fifty-five than men. Drilling down into the stats, cardiovascular disease accounts for around 22 per cent of all male deaths under the age of fifty-four, and 18.5 per cent of women. But once we get past fifty-five, the trend is reversed, with cardiovascular disease accounting for 38.5 per cent of male deaths and 41 per cent of female.[69] By the time we get to the age of eighty, our risk of CVD is about the same as that of men.[70] Heart disease is not a male disease! Please don't ever think that heart disease doesn't affect women. What's clear is that women typically develop heart disease later than men, which has led doctors to hypothesise that this is linked to the timing of the menopause transition.[71] Women tend to develop heart disease after the age of sixty, whereas with men it's after the age of fifty. This is precisely why our power decade is so important: we have a window post-menopause to look after our hearts.

Further research has found that women are less likely to seek medical attention when they experience discomfort or tightness in the chest, particularly because the acute chest pain we believe to be the main symptom of a heart attack can be absent when women experience cardiac issues. A study published early in 2022 found that, of over 200 patients treated for heart attacks in New York hospitals, 62 per cent of women did not have any chest pain or discomfort, compared to just 36 per cent of men.[72] The research team found that women were less likely to seek help because their symptoms didn't match their perceptions of what a heart attack could be, and they had to wait longer to be treated. Symptoms that can herald a female heart attack, such as shortness of breath, cold sweats, fatigue, and jaw and back pain, can often be attributed to other causes. Don't wait to seek help if you are concerned.

It's hard to overestimate the importance of looking after our hearts, but there is much we can do to make a huge difference to heart health in our fifties and sixties.

THE LINK BETWEEN HEART DISEASE AND REPRODUCTIVE HORMONES

Oestrogen acts like a lubricant for our endothelium, the cell-deep lining of our hearts, blood vessels and lymphatic system. This lining helps keep our blood vessels flexible and mobile and prevents the stiffening of the arteries linked to heart disease.[73]

Research tracking women across the menopause transition shows that higher levels of oestrogen (specifically, estradiol) equate to less narrowing of the arteries over time. The vasomotor symptoms of menopause (like hot flushes and night sweats) have been linked to increased risk of stiffened arteries. A meta-analysis looking at data from over 200,000 women found that those who reported menopause symptoms like hot flushes had an increased risk of cardio-vascular disease.[74]

In addition, low oestrogen post-menopause can contribute to raised cholesterol levels, which in turn impacts our heart health. For women who've experienced premature or early menopause, the risks are greater, simply because they've lost the protection of oestrogen earlier.

OTHER CAUSES OF HEART HEALTH ISSUES

Inflammation

As outlined on page 243, inflammation is at the root of so many of the chronic diseases of ageing. Combine that with the loss of the oestrogen that we know protects our arteries and we risk unhappy hearts. Inflammation drives the build-up of atherosclerosis, those fatty plaques that form on the walls of blood vessels, potentially blocking them. When inflammation is chronic rather than acute, it can start to cause damage to our blood vessels. If the lining of our arteries gets damaged, the immune system sends in the cavalry to repair the problem. That's acute inflammation. But if that damage is long term, for example if those cells suffer ongoing damage from high blood pressure, then the immune system goes into a constant state of repair, or chronic inflammation. It's this inflammation that can result in the build-up of fatty plaques on the artery wall, and thus cardiovascular disease.

Sleep

We know that menopause has a detrimental effect on sleep quality, and post-menopausal women are more likely to struggle to stay asleep than those who are pre-menopausal.[75] Research published in 2020 revealed that older adults with irregular sleep patterns – meaning that they have no regular schedule of sleeping and waking, or get varying amounts of sleep each night – are nearly twice as likely to develop cardiovascular disease.[76] The research found that the more irregular the sleep pattern, the more likely the study participants were to have CVD on a five-year follow-up. Go to the sleep chapter on page 111 to find out how to power up your sleep.

Cholesterol levels

Issues with heart disease and elevated cholesterol levels are one of the (many) points where ageing and the impact of declining reproductive hormones coincide. Sometimes it's difficult to tell which has the bigger impact on our health. But we do know that declining oestrogen levels result in higher cholesterol levels: one study found that levels of LDL (the so-called 'bad cholesterol') rose by 9 per cent in the two years around the final menstrual period.[77] Further research revealed that total cholesterol was much higher in post-menopausal women, but levels of HDL ('good cholesterol') were lower.[78]

Cholesterol is synthesised in the liver and is transported around the body, building cell membranes, creating hormones and making vitamin D. In charge of the transportation system are fatty molecules called lipoproteins – LDL carries cholesterol to our cells; HDL transports any excess back to the liver to be recycled. The process goes wrong when there's too much LDL in the body and it builds up in the walls of our blood vessels, causing them to narrow. Our friend, oestrogen, helps regulate the metabolism of these substances in the liver, so when it declines, LDL and triglycerides rise, increasing our risk of heart disease.

High blood pressure (hypertension)

Narrowing of the arteries in turn raises blood pressure, as our hearts must work harder to force blood through a small space. That increases systolic blood pressure (the higher number when you have your blood pressure tested), which reflects the force of the blood as it's pushed along by each heartbeat. The other number we're given in a blood pressure reading – diastolic pressure – is the level of pressure when the heart is at rest, between beats.

Declining oestrogen also contributes to high blood pressure: oestrogen has a vasodilative effect, meaning that it helps blood vessels dilate to ease blood flow. It also improves levels of nitric oxide, a chemical that relaxes and widens blood vessels.

Stress

Researchers have long linked heart disease and stress. You know that feeling when someone gives you a sudden shock and you find yourself yelling, 'You nearly gave me a heart attack!'? Stress has a huge impact on our hearts, both in the short and long term. Acute stress gets our hearts beating faster so we're ready to fight or run. Long-term, or chronic, stress keeps up the pressure on our health, and our hearts, for months or years. Many studies have linked it to increased risk of cardiovascular disease, coronary disease and stroke. Perceived stress, workplace stress, social isolation and childhood trauma can all lead to the build-up of heart-damaging stress.

Researchers have delved into the mechanisms by which stress damages hearts.[79] It starts with the area of the brain that processes feelings like stress and fear, the amygdala. Higher activity in the amygdala – i.e. when we're under stress – leads to increased white blood cell production in bone marrow, which in turn contributes to inflammation in the arteries. Increased bone marrow activity and inflammation are associated with increased rates of cardiovascular disease.

POWER UP: SMALL DAILY HABITS FOR BETTER HEART HEALTH

MINDSET

Cultivate optimism

Cultivate optimism for good heart health! It might not seem obvious, but multiple studies have shown that a positive outlook and a sense of optimism correlate with a lower risk of heart disease.[80] Negative emotions trigger a stress response. With a positive outlook, we're more likely to use healthy coping mechanisms and look after our health in other ways too.

We can train our brains to be objective about negative thoughts. They're just thoughts – they're not 'us'. We can decide whether or not to believe them. Catching a negative or distressing thought, then thanking our mind for worrying and keeping us safe, helps put stressful thoughts into perspective. This process has been a game changer for me.

MEALS

Power up on potassium

Research published in summer 2022 showed that a diet high in potassium can help lower blood pressure and thus protect women's hearts. A large-scale cohort study tracked the diets of women, with an average age of fifty-eight, and found that higher potassium intake correlated with lower blood pressure.[81]

Foods high in potassium include:

- Banana
- Beans, peas and lentils
- Seafood
- Sweet potato

Go nuts

Walnuts, pistachios, pine nuts, pecans, macadamias, hazelnuts, Brazil nuts and almonds have all been linked to lower LDL cholesterol and triglycerides. Walnuts have also been linked to better blood-wall function. The experts recommend around 40g – a good handful – of nuts a day to reap the benefits.

Oats and barley

The cell walls of these whole grains contain high levels of beta glucans, a soluble fibre that binds to cholesterol and helps the body excrete any excess. Eating 3g of beta glucans a day has been shown to reduce cholesterol levels by 10 per cent.

The best vegetables for heart health

Beetroot: It's the high level of nitric oxide that makes beautiful beetroot a heart-healthy food.[82] This helps open blood vessels and lower systolic blood pressure. Low levels of nitric oxide in the body may increase hypertension and poor endothelial function.

Avocado: The mono-unsaturated fats in avocados have been linked to lower cholesterol levels and a lower risk of heart disease. They're also rich in potassium.

Tomato: Low levels of the antioxidant lycopene, which gives tomatoes their red colour, may increase the risk of heart attack and stroke. When fifty overweight, midlife women ate two tomatoes a day for a month, they increased their levels of good HDL cholesterol.[83]

Vitamin K2

This vitamin works with vitamin D3 (the 'sunshine vitamin') to move calcium out of the arteries, where it can harden and form plaques. They transport it to the bones, where it's actually needed. This helps lower the risk of cardiovascular disease. It's not the easiest vitamin to find – most sources are animal ones, like meat, fatty fish, hard cheeses and eggs. It's also found in fermented foods like sauerkraut and kimchi. I take a combined D3 and K2 supplement in spray form.

Wise up on nutrition if you dine alone

It's hard if you live by yourself, but post-menopausal women who regularly eat alone have been found to have increased risk of cardiovascular disease.[84] They were also less know-ledgeable about nutrition, so keep learning and use this book to support you!

DASH

Dietary Approaches to Stop Hypertension, or the DASH diet for short, was developed to treat high blood pressure (also known as hypertension) in the States. It focuses on vegetables, pulses, whole grains, fruit and lean meat. It's also low in salt.

Salt

It's easy to overeat salt if we consume too many processed or snack foods. If you're cooking at home, you're unlikely to eat anything like the amount of salt found in fast food. Salt your food wisely and use a sea salt or Celtic salt if you can.

MOVEMENT

Cardiovascular exercise

The clue's in the name, so it makes sense that cardiovascular exercise is good for cardiovascular health. Government guidelines suggest a minimum of 150 minutes per week of moderate exercise, like brisk walking, or seventy-five minutes of high-intensity workouts, like running, cycling or a gym class. But there's really no upper limit to how much exercise we can do, if we want to.

Cardio helps control blood pressure because a healthy heart can push out more blood with each beat, allowing it to work more efficiently. This improved blood flow helps both the heart and small blood vessels where fatty deposits can build up. Better circulation in these areas reduces the risk of heart attacks.

When we get breathless, we're training our bodies to pull oxygen from our blood more efficiently, so our hearts learn to perform better under stress, we recover more quickly after exercise and our fitness increases.

Almost all exercise is good for the heart; it's being sedentary that is the problem. Anything that gets your heart pumping and results in a little breathlessness is good. The important thing is doing it consistently. What can you schedule in? Where does movement fit into your daily life? You will have heard these things before, but taking the stairs, parking further from your destination, and getting off the bus a stop earlier all add up to more heart-healthy activity per day.

We know that decreasing oestrogen levels may make us more sedentary, so we need to counteract that with a conscious effort to move more. New habits take time to bed in, which is why scheduling and planning well make such a difference.

Increase muscle mass

Also called resistance exercise, strength training has a specific impact on body composition – building lean muscle mass and reducing fat. In addition, the heart is a muscle, so exercising strengthens it, just like any other muscle. And building muscle throughout the body has a positive impact on heart health.[85] In fact, strength training may be even better for heart health than dynamic exercise like walking, running and cycling. Research that examined the heart health of 4,000 people found that those who did strength training had a reduced risk of cardiovascular disease compared to those who did cardio workouts. And the people who did best of all? The ones who did both.[86]

Find a way to strength train that suits you, and your fitness level, two to three times a week. It could be working out with hand weights (start small and build up over time), fixed weight machines at the gym or body-resistance exercises like squats, lunges and push-ups (for the latter, start on your knees or standing and leaning on a wall).

Raise nitric oxide levels

Nitric oxide is a molecule that's produced naturally by the body, aided by oestrogen, which keeps levels high pre-menopause. It helps the lining of blood vessels, the endothelium, to relax so our circulation works more effectively – a process called vasodilation. Eating vegetables high in nitrates, like beetroot, celery and lettuce, helps to restore levels post-menopause, as their nitrates are converted into nitric oxide in the body.

Breathe

All forms of exercise that get your blood pumping increase production of nitric oxide.

We also produce nitric oxide in the nasal cavity when we breathe through our nose. When we breathe through our mouth, we don't get the same benefits. Focus on slow, calm breathing through the nose whenever you can.

Get outside

Exposing our skin to the sun helps to create nitric oxide in the body. The sun helps convert nitrate in our skin cells to nitric oxide, which in turn increases vasodilation. Exercise outside for double benefits. When participants in a study by Edinburgh University were exposed to UV lamps, their blood pressure dropped significantly for an hour afterwards.[87] And it seems it was the nitric oxide that made the difference, not Vitamin D, as their vitamin D levels didn't increase.

Vitamin D

Vitamin D is important for heart health in other ways, however, and our skin synthesises it when exposed to the sun. Low levels of this vitamin have been linked to increased risk of developing cardiovascular disease.[88]

Be sensible about sun exposure, of course – no one wants sunburn. And sun exposure is a risk factor for skin cancer. But we've become so frightened of letting those rays hit our skin that we may be missing out on the incredible health-boosting benefits of the sun.

Try exposing your shoulders, neck or décolletage to create vitamin D in the body early in the morning or as the sun starts to sink in the sky. And even if you live in a country where the sky is perpetually grey and cloudy (as I do), fear not. UV rays penetrate the cloud and have a beneficial impact on nitric oxide and vitamin D levels, at least for part of the year.

Take a sauna

While most of us don't have access to a sauna on a regular basis, it's worth considering if your gym has one. Sauna bathing and exercise have both, individually, been found to support heart health. But follow a workout with a fifteen-minute sauna session and the benefits to blood pressure and heart health increase.[89]

DOES HRT HELP REDUCE HEART DISEASE RISK?

The Women's Health Initiative, the 2002 study that threw up concerns about the health risks of HRT and led to a generation of women not taking it, raised red flags not just about the increased risk of breast cancer for those on HRT, but also cardiovascular disease. Now, not only has that research been found to be flawed, it seems that the opposite is true. Re-evaluation of that research, and more recent studies, have shown that when HRT treatment is begun early enough, it can have a beneficial impact on the risk of coronary heart disease.[90]

'Early enough' needs definition, of course. Research that gave over 600 healthy post-menopausal women HRT for five years found that those who began the therapy within six years of their final menstrual period had less of the stiffening of the arteries associated with atherosclerosis than the control group. However, in

---

women who were ten or more years post-menopause, there was little benefit.[91]

A study by the university of Oslo in 2019 found that when post-menopausal women with a history of venous thrombosis were given HRT, their levels of LDL were reduced.[92]

However, in the UK, the British Menopause Society guidance to doctors is that HRT is only prescribed for symptom relief. Dr Carys Sonnenberg adds, 'Evidence shows that HRT, if started under the age of sixty, or within ten years of menopause, reduces the risk of cardiovascular disease and HRT will also protect the bones from osteoporosis.'

Boost Bone Health

To thrive post-menopause, we need to look after the skeleton that supports us, that literally holds us in place in this world. Our bones need to be strong to power us through this decade and beyond. It wasn't until I started writing about ageing well that I realised our bones are living, growing things! I thought they stopped growing when we did. How wrong I was – our bones evolve, with old bone tissue continually breaking down to be replaced with new. When too much old bone is broken down, or too little new bone is made, our bones weaken and we may find ourselves on the road to osteoporosis.

When I surveyed followers of The Age-Well Project about their health post-menopause, declining bone strength was the second biggest fear (after dementia). We're all conscious of the trips and falls, the broken wrists and hips that accompany so many women into older age. And we're right to be worried: over one third of White and Asian women will experience osteoporosis (literally: porous bones) in their lifetime, and most of those will suffer a fracture at some point. Black women have a lower prevalence of osteoporosis but face health disparities that put them at high risk of complications. Of those women who suffer a hip fracture, half won't be able to return to the lifestyle they had before. And women have four times the rate of osteoporosis than men.

Osteoporosis is known as 'the silent disease' because it can creep up on us unseen and unfelt, until a sudden fracture uncovers it. Osteopenia is the first stage of deteriorating bone density and can be diagnosed by a scan. Ask your doctor if you're concerned or have a family history of osteopenia or osteoporosis.

Our bones reach peak density in our late twenties, and then decline after the grand old age of thirty-five.[93] Not everyone is affected by a decline in bone density, but for some women, their bones will weaken most dramatically in the five to ten years after menopause and primary osteoporosis could kick in.[94] So, again, we need to make the most of this power decade to keep our bones resilient and put in place the behaviours that will help keep us out of the fracture clinic as we age.

THE LINK BETWEEN BONE STRENGTH AND REPRODUCTIVE HORMONES

The accelerated loss of bone density before and after the menopause transition is linked, of course, to the decline of our protective pal, oestrogen. In addition to all its other roles,

oestrogen regulates bone metabolism, that process of breaking down and rebuilding bone tissue so it can stay strong.

Before the start of perimenopause, we lose around 0.13 per
cent of bone density annually. During perimenopause,
that decline can ramp up to 2.5 per cent a year – a huge
acceleration – and stay at that level until we're about sixty,
when it tapers off.

Progesterone and testosterone also have roles to play,
promoting bone formation and increasing bone turnover.
To understand how reproductive hormones regulate bone
strength, we need to grasp the idea that our bones are not
solid structures. They're essentially a matrix – a 3-D mesh of
proteins and minerals. Over 90 per cent of this matrix is
made up of osteocytes, mature cells that are buried in the
mineral matrix of bone. The rest of our bone is osteoblasts
– which birth new bone cells – and osteoclasts, our skeleton's
recycling service, reabsorbing or breaking down bone.

Our reproductive hormones support the work of all three
types of bone cell in maintaining proper bone formation.
When levels drop, the cycle of creating and breaking down
bone becomes disrupted, with bone formation slowing
and bone resorption increasing.[95] And this in turn leads to
cavities developing in the bone, making them 'porous', less
able to support our weight and more likely to fracture.

OTHER CAUSES OF BONE WEAKENING

Sedentary behaviour

Bones need movement in order to remodel and rebuild. And yet by the time we reach the age of sixty-five, we're likely to be sitting for around ten hours a day. Exercise, particularly the loading that comes with weight-bearing exercise, stimulates new bone formation. And if we don't exercise, we lose muscle too, meaning that there's both greater wear and tear on our bones, and less of the push and pull that comes from the action of muscle on bone.

Alcohol and smoking

Alcohol impacts how well we absorb calcium and vitamin D, both of which are crucial for healthy bones. Calcium is absorbed via the intestine, whereas vitamin D is metabolised via the pancreas, but both are affected by alcohol. Nicotine from cigarettes attaches itself to osteoblasts, eventually killing them off. Smoking can increase the risk of osteoporosis by up to a third.

Lack of sunlight

Sunlight is one of the most potent forces we have at our disposal: we evolved to harness its power for our health. But now we spend the vast majority of our days indoors, under artificial, junky light, which harms our health. It's one of the great travesties of the modern world. The vitamin D we make in our skin from sunlight helps us absorb and use calcium, the raw material of new bone. From October to March we don't get enough sunlight in the UK to make vitamin D, so we need to get it in supplemental form.

Caffeine

There are lots of ways that caffeine is good for our health – it's been linked to better cognition, for example – but a caffeine intake of over 300mg per day (there's around 100mg in a 330ml/12oz cup of regular coffee) has been linked to increased excretion of calcium and interferes with vitamin D absorption. Research has shown a higher fracture risk among women who consume four or more cups of coffee per day, especially in those having less than 700mg of calcium daily.[96]

POWER UP: SMALL DAILY HABITS TO KEEP BONES STRONG

MINDSET

Understand what you want to achieve

I talked to Rebekah Rotstein of Buff Bones®, who has worked with The Royal Osteoporosis Society. She explained that if we want strong bones, we don't just want them to be hard, we want them to be flexible as well, which accounts for their resiliency to resist fracture. 'Your goal is not to have high bone density,' she explains. 'Your goal is to not fracture and to live an independent life. We need to avoid falls because falls are what lead to fractures. You do this by strengthening your bones and your body. But you also need to maintain and improve your balance and responsiveness to avoid falls, because falls lead to fractures. Along with this, you need to improve alignment, posture and mobility.'

Let's get past the mindset that we just need our bones to be 'dense'; instead we need to get our minds working to create a life in which we don't get fractures. Rebekah goes on to explain, 'Your bone health exercise regimen should give you all the elements you need to move effectively, to avoid injury, to avoid falls and to avoid fractures and to live an active, fulfilling life.'

MEALS

Calcium

Calcium intake provides the raw materials for bone turnover. We need 700mg of calcium daily (that's the Nutrient Reference Value, i.e. the recommended daily intake in the UK. In the USA it's 1,200mg for women over fifty, in Australia and New Zealand it's 1,300mg). Calcium-rich foods, like dairy products, sardines (buy the cheap tinned ones with the bones!), and soy products, like tofu and green leafy vegetables, are all good calcium sources.

- 100g canned sardines with bones = 351mg calcium
- 100g tofu = 351mg calcium

- 100g Greek yogurt = 110mg calcium
- 100g spinach = 99mg calcium
- 200ml semi-skimmed milk = 248mg calcium
- 100g Parmesan cheese = 1100mg calcium

Vitamins D3 and K2

These two vitamins work together to move calcium from our blood to our bones, i.e. from where we don't want it to where we do. Get dietary vitamin D from oily fish and eggs. Most people need at least 600 international units (IU) of vitamin D a day. That recommendation increases to 800 IU a day after age seventy. K2 is found in meat (particularly liver), eggs and dairy products. Plant-based sources include sauerkraut, kimchi and a fermented soy product called natto, which I'm afraid I find absolutely disgusting!

Magnesium

Around 60 per cent of the magnesium in our bodies is stored in our bones and it plays a crucial role in preventing osteoporosis. In a seven-year study of post-menopausal women, a higher intake of magnesium was associated with greater bone-mineral density.[97]

Get magnesium from almonds, avocados, bananas, beans, broccoli, green leafy vegetables, nuts and seeds, fish, whole grains, soy and dark chocolate.

MOVEMENT

Don't be afraid to move

In the past there's been a reluctance by healthcare professionals to prescribe higher intensity exercise for women with low bone mass because of the risk of fracture or other injury. But a study published in the *Journal of Bone and Mineral Research* found that thirty minutes of well-supervised, high-intensity resistance training twice a week improved bone health in post-menopausal women, without injury.[98] However, take advice from a healthcare professional before you introduce any new exercise.

Create a combination of exercise

One form of exercise alone is not enough to keep bones healthy and fracture-free. We need to combine weight-bearing exercise such as walking, jogging, running, stair climbing and skipping rope with strength training using weights or body weight, as well as balance exercises.

Power up posture

No amount of exercise will undo the damage of bad posture for multiple hours a day. Sit or stand as tall as possible, shoulders back and down, stomach gently pulled in. Check yourself in a mirror and stick a Post-it note somewhere you see regularly with the words 'Don't slouch' written on it!

Strengthen hip muscles

Strong hip muscles will help prevent fracture by cushioning the hips and improving alignment. Try a glute bridge: lying on your back on the floor, feet on the ground and knees bent at a ninety-degree angle, lift your hips towards the ceiling and squeeze your buttock muscles. Lower gently to the ground and repeat. A 'psoas hold' works in a similar way but also engages balance. Standing straight – with something nearby to grab on to if necessary – lift one knee above ninety degrees and try to keep it there for a few seconds.

Kyphosis exercises

Kyphosis refers to curvature of the spine linked to loss of bone mass, and is a risk for post-menopausal women. Working on bone and muscle strength will help reduce that risk. Rebekah advocates lying down on the floor face up first thing in the morning with knees bent to unweight the spine. From that position, try slowly sweeping your arms in an arc as if you're making angel wings while you breathe mindfully, to open up the shoulders. To strengthen the back, lie face down with your arms by your side. From that position, lift your head, hands and shoulders off the ground without lifting your chest and feet, while still looking down. Build endurance as you go along.

Boost balance

You've probably heard the 'brush your teeth standing on one leg' trick, haven't you? Rebekah urges us to work on our balance in different ways, standing on one leg but extending the endurance so we do it for longer. Could you stand on one leg and move your limbs, turn your head, close your eyes? How can you push this a little further? She also suggests standing on one leg on different surfaces, such as a carpet or padded mat rather than a wooden floor for additional challenge.

DOES HRT HELP KEEP BONES STRONG?

NOGG, the National Osteoporosis Guideline Group for the UK, recommends HRT for the treatment of post-menopausal osteoporosis for women under sixty who have low baseline risk for cancer and heart disease. The British Menopause Society has also stated that HRT offers protection against fractures of the hips and spine.

Dr Juliet Balfour pointed out to me that, when/if you stop HRT, you lose both the cardiovascular and bone benefits. If you are on HRT for the treatment of osteoporosis and you're planning to come off it, it is important to talk to your GP or specialist about starting alternative medication to support bone health.

Build a Better Brain

My journey into my own power decade began with the determination to keep my brain as happy and healthy as I can, for as long as possible. My mother's dementia diagnosis was a turning point for me in terms of my own health: being responsible for her for twelve years opened my eyes to the impact of this condition on the whole family.

When I surveyed followers of The Age-Well Project about their biggest health concern post-menopause, fear of dementia was the number-one issue. In my own coaching practice, I help women work to reduce their risk of dementia. I see that fear over and over, particularly among those who, like me, have cared for a loved one with Alzheimer's.

And we're right to be fearful: here in the UK, dementia is now the leading cause of death,[99] and worldwide it's seventh. Women are twice as likely to suffer dementia as men, and that's not due to living longer. Alzheimer's is a women's disease – we are more likely to get it and more likely to care for others who have it.

We consider Alzheimer's to be a disease of old age, but in reality the changes in our brains that precipitate the disease start to develop twenty to thirty years earlier. With most diagnoses happening between the ages of sixty-five and eighty, that puts the starting point for those brain changes somewhere between our mid-forties and late fifties. Which is also the time that something else happens too. What was it again? Oh, yes, menopause. And that means the time to address our brain health is now, in our fifties and sixties, to reduce our risk of adding to those statistics.

My own training as a coach with Dr Dale Bredesen, the American neuroscientist and author of *The End of Alzheimer's Programme*, has shown me that there's so much we can do to keep our brains strong and healthy in our fifties, sixties and beyond.

A paper published in 2020 reveals that around 40 per cent of dementia cases are attributable to lifestyle factors. We really can make a difference to our brain health.[100]

THE LINK BETWEEN BRAIN HEALTH AND REPRODUCTIVE HORMONES

It's not surprising that brain function is impacted during menopause: nowhere is the idea that oestrogen, progesterone and testosterone are merely hormones of reproduction less true than when it comes to our brains. Menopause changes our brain chemistry in a fundamental way.

There are oestrogen receptors throughout the brain, and when levels of that hormone diminish, the structure of the brain alters, energy metabolism falters and beta amyloid deposits (a sticky plaque linked to Alzheimer's) increase. Without the neuroprotective benefits of oestrogen, the brain is more vulnerable to ageing and decline. Testosterone also plays a role in brain development and function.

Scans of women's brains before and after menopause show a frightening reduction in the amount of activity, a decline of up to 30 per cent in a relatively short time, and that's for cognitively normal women.[101] If you want to know more, look at the brilliant work of Dr Lisa Mosconi, author of *The XX Brain*. Her website has clear illustrations and explanations of this process (lisamosconi.com). She refers to menopause as 'a dynamic neurological transition' and it's not hard to see why. As she points out, menopause impacts the brain as much as it does the ovaries.

There are oestrogen receptors in parts of the brain, like the hippocampus and prefrontal cortex, which are involved with learning and memory.[102] The hypothalamus controls the sleep-wake cycle. When it doesn't get the oestrogen it needs, sleep becomes more difficult. Sound familiar? And what about the amygdala, which regulates emotions? When that doesn't get enough oestrogen, we experience mood swings. Menopausal symptoms really are the result of diminishing hormones in our brain.

But the good news is that, in terms of day-to-day function, our brains find a new normal post-menopause. Dr Fionnuala Barton explains, 'During menopause the brain is changing, in the same way our brains change and remodel themselves during adolescence. But what the brain research is suggesting is that, actually, we're pruning the neurons that we don't need any more and, when we come out of menopause, our brains are more efficient in some ways because we've lost pathways we don't necessarily need.'

Post-menopause, grey matter volume and brain biomarkers recover.[103] Energy metabolism steadies, brain fog should recede. Our brains seem to be able to adapt and overcome. Just as we do.

OTHER CAUSES OF POOR BRAIN HEALTH

Ageing

Cognitive decline isn't solely a women's issue, nor is it simply a hormonal one. Ageing impacts the brain regardless of hormonal status. So often, our lives are not geared to optimising a healthy brain. And we don't think about our brains enough – we need to keep them front of mind, as it were!

Ageing also brings with it microvascular changes in the brain, which can ultimately give rise to vascular dementia and cause cognitive issues in later life.

Stress

Stress is the enemy of a well-functioning brain. Engaging in 'stress-related unconstructive repetitive thought' (psychology-speak for overthinking) negatively affects the brain in the short and long term. Short term, it's linked to a shorter attention span and worse cognitive performance day-to-day; long term, stress results in accelerated cognitive decline.[104]

Women under stress have much lower levels of a hormone called klotho, which regulates ageing and enhances cognition. This hormone seems to be the link between chronic stress and reduced life expectancy.

The stressed brain shunts resources that could be used to lay down memories into managing stress in the amygdala, the emotional centre of the brain. That stress pushes the brain into survival mode rather than memory mode.[105] Being under stress like this in the long term is linked to a higher risk of Alzheimer's.

Sugars and simple carbs

The insulin rollercoaster initiated by sugars and simple carbs, like white bread and plain pasta, is as bad for our brain as it is for our waistline. Our brains are greedy, burning around 20 per cent of our daily energy requirement, despite being just 3 per cent of our bodies by volume. So one fifth of what we consume is going straight to our brains. A –

literally – sobering thought. And a very useful reminder of the importance of the quality of our nutritional intake. Our greedy brains use glucose as their primary fuel, but, as we get older, and particularly once the oestrogen receptors in the brain power down, they don't use that fuel as effectively as they once did.

Environmental toxins

We live in a toxic world. Air pollution has recently been recognised as one of the modifiable risk factors for Alzheimer's disease. We can't individually solve the issue of poor air quality, but we can do all we can to minimise our exposure, and maximise our detoxification. Dr Dale Bredesen, with whom I trained, has coined the term 'dementogens' to describe chemicals associated with dementia, just as carcinogens are chemicals associated with cancer. Metals like mercury and lead, chemicals in cleaning products and pesticides, and biotoxins from damp and mould all fall into this category.

Poor sleep

It's during deep sleep that our brains carry out their daily housekeeping, sweeping out toxins that have accumulated during the day. Our brilliant brain cells can shrink up to 60 per cent while we sleep so that the glymphatic system – the brain's housekeeping team – can get to work. But if we're not getting that quality sleep, the deep clean doesn't happen and toxins related to Alzheimer's can accumulate. That, in turn, creates a cascade effect, with the build-up of amyloid beta plaques associated with Alzheimer's making deep sleep more difficult. And it's during sleep that our brains process the huge amount of information they encounter during the day, filing and storing information to create memories – if we don't sleep well, that process can't happen.

Lack of stimulation

Our brains love novelty, and thrive on building new neural connections throughout our lives. It used to be thought that our brains remained the same size, or shrank, in adulthood, but more recent research has shown that they can create new neurons if we give them the stimulation. But that's the critical point: if they don't get stimulated, it's a downward slope. We need to give our brains the opportunity to grow, learn and adapt – a process called neuroplasticity.

POWER UP: SMALL DAILY HABITS FOR BETTER BRAIN HEALTH

MINDSET

Think about your brain

We need to love our brains! We spend all day using our brains to think, but we don't think about our brains enough. Nothing will make a bigger difference to our experience of the power decade than a healthy brain. We want to use this time to keep our cognition sharp, to ensure that our brain is in good shape to keep us happy as well as healthy. Good brain health and good mental health are so closely intertwined that we can't have one without the other. Ask yourself if the decisions you make each day are good for your brain, or not?

Seek novelty

Staying curious about the world throughout our power decade is crucial to keeping our brains wiring and firing. Any new experience is good: that can be setting off on a world tour or taking a new route to work. Anything that challenges our brains with newness makes a difference. Our brains create habits to reduce their workload, but anything that challenges those habits helps create new neurons.

Follow your passion

Life-long learning is an obvious – and important – way to develop neuroplasticity. That doesn't mean going back to school – although that's great – but learning in new ways too: podcasts, webinars, language classes and music lessons all work. Find something you're passionate about and pursue it. Getting absorbed in a hobby is an effective way to both relax and stimulate the brain.

Build a support network

The strength and breadth of our social connections help determine our health throughout our lives. We may well find ourselves going through a period of intense changes during the power decade: empty nest, redundancy, relationship breakdown. These can all shake our connections to their foundations and leave us wondering who's really there for us. We need to be able to answer that question. A strong support system almost halves our dementia risk and has a profound effect on our longevity. Your life experiences may have changed you, your goals may have changed – ask yourself if your social support network has kept up?

Meditate

I use the simple but powerful practice of Kirtan Kriya meditation to help recharge my brain and reduce stress. It's part of the kundalini yoga system, and has been shown to increase blood flow to the brain and reduce biomarkers linked to Alzheimer's.[106] It isn't the type of yoga where you just sit quietly. The practice involves chanting and finger movements, which can feel a bit silly until you get used to it. But the good thing is that you really need to focus so your mind can't wander! You need to listen to a guide as you chant; I use a free YouTube video by Nina Mongendre, with music by Nirinjan Kaur. It's just eleven minutes long and I feel so much better when I've done it.

MEALS

The MIND diet

The brilliantly named MIND diet, which stands for the slightly less snappy Mediterranean-DASH Intervention for Neurodegenerative Delay, has been shown to reduce dementia risk. The diet suggests ten foods to eat:

- Green leafy vegetables
- All other vegetables
- Berries
- Nuts
- Olive oil
- Whole grains
- Fish
- Beans
- Poultry
- Wine (but only in tiny amounts!)

And five foods to avoid:

- Butter and margarine
- Cheese
- Red meat
- Fried food
- Pastries and sweets

Cut out sugar and ultra-processed foods

Sugar and ultra-processed foods have no place in a brain-healthy diet. They provide none of the nutrition our greedy brains need, and send us on a toxic rollercoaster of sugar crashes. Focus on whole foods, plenty of vegetables and unprocessed proteins and your brain will thank you.

SMASH fish

Our brains love the omega-3 fatty acids EPA and DHA, which provide them with a particularly rich form of fuel. Feed them oily fish, remembering the acronym SMASH: salmon, mackerel, anchovies, sardines and herring.

Berries, greens, greens

This is the mantra that my clients tell me sticks more than any other! I use it as a simple reminder that each meal can help support our brain health. If we make sure that berries are part of breakfast, and we add greens to our other two meals, we're on our way to creating a way of eating that supports our brain health throughout the power decade.

Tea, but make it green

What we drink is as important for our brain as what we eat. Staying properly hydrated, and adding green tea to our daily drinks roster, makes a huge difference. Green tea is packed with the polyphenol EGCG, which research shows helps protect the brain from oxidation and increases the production of dopamine, one of the 'feelgood' hormones.

Nuts nuts nuts

Nuts are nutritional powerhouses for our brains, providing healthy fats, fibre and protein in neat little packages. And the best nut for brain health? It's no coincidence walnuts are shaped like tiny brains! They're packed full of an omega-3 fatty acid called alpha-linolenic acid and polyphenols to help reduce inflammation.

What even are healthy fats?

Our brains are essentially balls of fat and water, so we need to keep them fuelled with both. Energy from fats like olive oil, avocado and nuts doesn't spike our insulin and provides our brains with a steady fuel supply.

If you can, fast

On page 252, I discuss why intermittent fasting, or time-restricted eating, is not for everyone, particularly if you're experiencing menopausal symptoms. It can leave us too depleted and stressed to be beneficial. But when it comes to brain health, a short period of not eating can allow both body and brain to rest and repair. Digestion is hard work for the body, so it stands to reason that it's not able to repair while it's digesting. Research has shown that fasting improves brain function and emotional wellbeing.[107]

MOVEMENT

Just move

Exercise is the most heavily researched brain booster there is. The process of neurogenesis – creating new brain cells – happens when we exercise. As does the production of brain-derived neurotrophic factor (BDNF), a kind of Miracle-Gro for brain cells. But we need to think beyond short bursts of exercise and work as much movement as we can into our lives every day. It would be wonderful if there was one exercise that could improve brain health, but life is never that simple. We need a mixture of daily low-intensity movement plus strength training, aerobic and mind-body exercises to power up our brains.

Bounce!

It's not for everyone, but rebounding – bouncing on a small trampoline – has been linked to better brain health (it's also fun!). It helps activate the lymphatic system, a network of tissues and organs that helps rid the body of waste and toxins. This system transports lymph, a fluid containing infection-fighting white blood cells, round the body. Lymph is entirely dependent on our physical movement (unlike blood, which has the heart to pump it). Rebounding helps get lymph flowing.

Walk and then walk some more

Regular walks change the structure of our brains, developing the prefrontal cortex, which in turn improves memory and concentration. Walking improves blood flow and oxygenation of the brain, so both cognitive function and mood are improved. The – very specific! – target of 8,900 steps a day has been found to improve brain health.

Build leg strength

Studies have shown a clear correlation between strong leg muscles and greater brain power. It seems that weight-bearing exercise, like walking, dancing and running, sends an instruction to the brain to create healthy neurons.[108]

HRT AND THE BRAIN

You may have heard suggestions that HRT can reduce the risk of Alzheimer's and vascular dementia, but at the moment there's not enough evidence to prove this. Dr Juliet Balfour explains, 'In theory, because we know HRT reduces inflammation and atherosclerosis in blood vessels, we think HRT could reduce the risk of vascular dementia – but we haven't got the evidence yet. We just don't know enough about Alzheimer's but research is ongoing. So with Alzheimer's, as with all dementias, looking at your lifestyle is important to reduce your risk.'

Research by Dr Roberta Diaz Brinton (who works closely with Dr Lisa Mosconi) found a positive association between HRT and lower Alzheimer's risk. She studied ten years' worth of medical insurance records from almost 400,000 women over the age of forty-five and found that those who'd taken HRT at the time of menopause lowered their risk of developing Alzheimer's and other neurodegenerative diseases later in life by 50 per cent.[109]

Douse Inflammation

Inflammation is so closely linked to ageing that scientists have coined the term 'inflammageing' to highlight the link. And almost all age-related diseases have inflammation as a starting point. So what is it, and why is it so damaging?

Acute inflammation is the product of our immune system, which sends it racing to the scene like an inbuilt paramedic when we're hurt – if we cut a finger, say, or contract a virus. That's a good thing, and once we've healed the inflammation goes away. But – and this is a big but – as we age, damaged cells build up in our bodies. Our immune system sees this build-up as a threat and responds with chronic, low-grade inflammation that never goes away. This kind of inflammation can be triggered by a low-quality diet or too much alcohol and stress, but also occurs naturally as we age. It's switched on by oxidation in our bodies (think: rust, but inside humans), the by-product of decades of turning food into fuel and burning oxygen just to stay alive. Once it's switched on, it stays on – and chronic inflammation can contribute to all the conditions of ageing.

We don't always know we have inflammation – we don't feel inflamed, but it's there. It can be one of the asymptomatic changes that happens in our bodies, and impacts our health, as we reach midlife. Inflammation is the root cause of many health issues like dementia, cardiovascular disease, diabetes and cancer, as well as inflammatory diseases like arthritis, all of which are most likely to emerge ten to fifteen years after the onset of menopause.

THE LINK BETWEEN INFLAMMATION AND REPRODUCTIVE HORMONES

As we pass through the menopause transition, our falling oestrogen levels can cause anti-inflammatory antibodies in the immune system to switch sides and become pro-inflammatory. There's a clear difference in inflammation levels pre- and post-menopause.

Research undertaken in Denmark and published in 2020 looked in detail at levels of inflammation in women aged between forty-five and sixty.[110] The women who were post-menopausal clearly had increased chronic systemic inflammation. They also had more senescent cells – damaged or dying 'zombie' cells that hang around pumping out more inflammation. This creates a vicious cycle of inflammation in the body: more inflammation, leading to more zombie cells, leading to more inflammation. Earlier research found that within five years of menopause, women had more inflammatory cytokines in their system.[111]

One review described the association of chronic inflammation with oestrogen decline, and their combined impact on our health, as 'posing major health challenges for twenty-first-century women'.[112]

OTHER CAUSES OF INFLAMMATION

Ageing

As we get older, we can't lay all the blame for inflammation, and inflammageing, at menopause's door. Let's face it, we've got a few decades under our belts by now, so inflammation is naturally building up in our bodies with age. There are many other causes of inflammation to consider: some we can tackle and some we need to mitigate against, because we can't eliminate them entirely.

The world around us

I hate to say this, but we live in an inflamed world. People are more divided and distrustful than ever before. We are surrounded by inflammatory opinions. Whenever we look at the news or social media, we're targeted by negativity, which is both inflammatory and ageing. Oppression is inflammatory; other people's anger is inflammatory. Conflict is inflammatory – it adds to our stress levels, which has a physical effect in our body over time.

Ultra-processed foods

Half of the food consumed in the UK is now considered ultra-processed. By ultra-processed, I mean products made in a factory with ingredients we're unlikely to have in our kitchens at home. They're full of scientific-sounding ingredients that may give them a long shelf-life and hyper-palatability (i.e. it's hard to stop eating them), but our bodies don't recognise them as food and respond as if they're a foreign body. Our immune system pumps out inflammation to deal with the invader, even if we've consumed it willingly . . .

Stress

There's a very close correlation between stress and inflammation. When we are stressed, inflammation rises, and when we relax, it lowers. One study looked at 600 people in middle age and beyond and found a close correlation between money worries and inflammation.[113] We all handle stress differently and we all handle inflammation differently. Inflammation has a direct impact not just on our bodies, but on our brains too: people suffering with depression often have high levels of inflammation. Stress also has a very direct impact on the strength – the integrity – of our gut wall, more on which below.

Leaky gut

Our gut wall is all that stands between us and everything we ingest. It's only one cell thick – that's tiny! Leaky gut is a condition in which the lining of the small intestine becomes damaged, causing undigested food particles, toxic waste products and bacteria to 'leak' through the intestines and flood the bloodstream, causing inflammation. The gut is highly susceptible to stress, and, post-menopause, the make-up of our gut microbiota shifts, leaving us with more inflammatory bacteria.

Lack of exercise

Physical activity can reduce inflammation, so it stands to reason that lack of exercise has the opposite effect. Exercise also boosts our immune system to deal with chronic inflammation. Our white blood cells are sedentary, so we literally need to shake them up to get them moving round our bodies. Research published at the end of 2021 showed that older adults who exercise more had less inflammation in the brain – and therefore a lower Alzheimer's risk.[114] The research team found it didn't matter what movement the study participants did, it was simply the amount of movement that counted.

A WORD ABOUT AUTOIMMUNE DISEASES

Autoimmune diseases, such as rheumatoid arthritis, lupus, inflammatory bowel disease, fibromyalgia, MS or psoriasis, are the result of the body's immune system attacking healthy tissues. This occurs when the immune system can no longer tell the difference between healthy cells and invading nasties, so it goes to war. This is different to the inflammageing I've talked about above, when the body is under pressure from lack of oestrogen, ageing cells and exterior factors.

Both issues, however, have links to the hormonal changes that come with the menopause transition. Around 78 per cent of those affected by autoimmune conditions are women.[115] Hormones interact with the immune system and inflammatory cytokines, and there's a delicate balance between them all. If one is out of whack, then the rest will be too. Research shows a strong link between hormonal transitions and the onset of auto-immune disease.

POWER UP: SMALL DAILY HABITS TO REDUCE INFLAMMATION

MINDSET

Feel good about yourself

Levels of dopamine, the body's reward system, are lowered by chronic inflammation. In turn, a hit of dopamine helps reduce inflammation in the body. A really easy way to raise dopamine levels is to start the day with a quick win. Any small activity that makes you feel good will work. It could be as simple as making your bed or doing a few stretches. A five-minute meditation, sitting quietly and focusing on your breath, can help lower inflammation.

Do what makes you happy

Seeking activities that make us happy reduces inflammation in the body. A study of 140 people with type 2 diabetes found that those who reported higher levels of daily happiness had lower levels of inflammation.[116] And if you think happiness is a rather vague term, then another study[117] asked its middle-aged participants about their daily experiences of sixteen positive emotions: enthusiastic, interested, determined, excited, amused, inspired, alert, active, strong, proud, attentive, happy, relaxed, cheerful, at ease and calm. They were also asked to rate whether they'd felt sixteen *negative* emotions: scared, afraid, upset, distressed, jittery, nervous, ashamed, guilty, irritable, hostile, tired, sluggish, sleepy, blue, sad and drowsy. The negative emotions didn't seem to affect levels of inflammation, but the range of positive emotions did. People who'd experienced a wide range of emotions – known as emodiversity – had the lowest levels of inflammation.

Celebrate your wins

In his fabulous book *Tiny Habits*, behaviourist B. J. Fogg exhorts us to celebrate our wins, however small, in order to create a positive feeling inside that he calls 'Shine'. Celebrating helps wire a habit into our brains. He suggests we

create our own celebration style and gives 100 examples –
some crazier than others – such as:

- Say 'Yes!' while you do a fist pump
- Visualise fireworks going off for you
- Throw imaginary confetti
- Strike a power pose
- Say 'You got this!'
- Inhale and think of energy entering you

Swerve the inflammatory world

We can't avoid the world around us, with its twenty-four-
hour news cycle and endless updates. But we can reduce
our interactions with the more stressful and inflammatory
elements of it. Review your daily experience of news, toxic
social media and any situation that makes you compare
yourself to others.

MEALS

Mostly Medi

The Mediterranean diet has been linked to reduced inflammation levels in multiple studies. Here's one in particular:
research published late in 2021 looked at the link between
inflammatory diets and the risk of dementia in older
individuals in Greece.[118] They found that those consuming
highly inflammatory diets were over three times more

likely to develop dementia than those consuming anti-inflammatory diets. I love this quote from the lead researcher, Dr Nikolaos Scarmeas, 'There may be some potent nutritional tools in your home to help fight the inflammation that could contribute to brain ageing.' The research found that the people consuming the most fruit, vegetables, beans, tea and coffee had the lowest inflammatory markers.

The zinc link

Of course, we need a wide range of vitamins and minerals to protect our cells and DNA from damage due to inflammation. Zinc, in particular, is essential, as it also helps us manage stress. We find it in foods such as meat, shellfish and pulses/beans.

The increased inflammation that happens as we age runs in parallel to decreasing zinc absorption, so we need to make sure we're getting enough. The UK recommended dietary allowance (RDA) is 7mg a day for women aged nineteen to sixty-four years.

As a side note, a randomised control trial (the gold standard for scientific research studies) found that post-menopausal women given zinc supplements had improved sexual function and desire, as well as reduced vaginal dryness.[119]

Work out how much zinc you're getting:

- 100g raw ground beef = 4.8 mg zinc
- 80g brown crab = 5.2mg zinc
- 100g dark meat turkey = 3.4mg zinc
- 100g cashews = 5.6mg zinc
- 100g hemp seeds = 10mg zinc
- 100g cooked lentils = 4.8mg zinc

Intermittent fasting

Not eating is as important as eating when it comes to reducing post-menopausal inflammation. A short period of overnight fasting, also known as time-restricted eating, lowers inflammation and improves longevity. The body goes into repair mode, activating inbuilt healing mechanisms designed to keep it alive when food is scarce.

A study found that fasting results in a lower level of the cells that cause inflammation – monocytes – in the blood.[120] It seems that eating all the time, without allowing our bodies to rest and digest, causes excess monocytes in the blood, which in turn creates more inflammation.

Omega-3 and -6

Studies consistently show a connection between high omega-3 intake and reduced inflammation. Load up on omega-3s from walnuts, flax seeds, chia seeds and particularly oily fish. The omega-3s in fish like salmon, mackerel and sardines, which are known as EPA and DHA, are particularly powerful inflammation busters.

Omega-6 fatty acids do vital work supporting cell membranes and are found in whole nuts and seeds, soya meat, fish and eggs. These are all great foods to be eating. Unfortunately, we also get a huge amount of omega-6 in our diet from fried foods and heavily processed vegetable oils. We need a balance of omega-3 and omega-6, so that omega-3 can work efficiently to reduce inflammation. But with too much omega-6 around, it doesn't work as effectively.

Check how much seed/vegetable oil you're consuming – it's found in a lot of 'healthy' foods, like oat milk! Also think about the oils you're using in your kitchen. I use olive oil for everything these days – an extra virgin one for dressings and drizzling, and a lighter one for cooking.

Polyphenols

Polyphenols are bioactive compounds found in plants that help fight inflammation in the body. Good sources include:

- Berries – the darker the better
- Pomegranate
- Blackcurrants – they have really high polyphenol levels!
- Herbs and spices, particularly cloves, turmeric and rosemary
- Cocoa powder
- Nuts and flax seeds
- Vegetables, especially artichokes, parsley, sprouts, chicory, red onions, spinach

- Olives and olive oil
- Coffee, tea, green tea

MOVEMENT

Keep active to lower inflammation levels

ALL exercise helps reduce inflammation, unless you do too much for too long. Overexercising can trigger production of the stress hormone cortisol. But research has shown that something as simple as a twenty-minute walk can have an anti-inflammatory effect.[121]

Flick through the movement section of this book and get out your diary. Block out time for any form of movement you want to do – schedule a walk, book an exercise class. Do whatever it takes to make it a non-negotiable in your diary.

A Note on Cancer Risk

Let's be clear: menopause doesn't cause cancer, but our risk does increase through our fifties and sixties. Why? Really, it's down to age. With breast cancer, for example, age is the single most important factor for increased risk: about 95 per cent of women diagnosed with breast cancer are over age forty, and half are over sixty-one. One in eight women in the UK will be given a breast cancer diagnosis during their lifetime, meaning all of us will know someone who has it.

Risks for colon, uterine, ovarian, vaginal and vulval cancers also increase with age. There can be a lifestyle element to our cancer risk, but some are genetically predetermined and our life experiences will influence how those genes are expressed. And as Dr Fionnuala Barton explains, we may have little influence over that in the early part of our lives. 'A lot of us haven't had the agency in our childhood years to impact what happens in terms of epigenetics. And we might only have woken up to the fact that we can influence our health and wellbeing outcomes in our thirties, forties or beyond.'

WHY DOES CANCER RISK INCREASE POST-MENOPAUSE?

Dr Barton explains, 'We know across the board that, with most cancers, if you can avoid things we know to be carcinogenic – smoking, poor diet, inactivity, alcohol – then you're going to have a slightly lower cancer risk. But we all know people with cancer who live incredibly healthy lives, so it isn't just about lifestyle. It's about something we don't have control over in many ways.'

So what is it about midlife that increases our risk? Dr Barton says, 'It's probably a huge combination of issues. I think that the cardiometabolic issues are bound to have an impact: if our cells aren't necessarily working as well as they should be to divide reliably, then we're at an increased risk of that cell division going wrong. And if that's going wrong repeatedly and that's forming a tumour somewhere, we have a problem.'

DOES HRT INCREASE MY CANCER RISK?

Broadly, no, but – as with so many other things – the answer isn't quite that simple.

We know that for a woman with a womb, oestrogen therapy needs to be combined with progesterone to reduce the risk of endometrial cancer, because oestrogen alone can cause a thickening of the endometrium (the lining of the womb), which can increase cancer risk. And there's a small increased risk of breast cancer associated with combined HRT (oestrogen and progesterone). But a bigger risk factor for both these cancers is being overweight.

HRT is rarely prescribed for women who have had, or have a high risk of, oestrogen-dependent breast cancer. Although it can be, for a short time, if symptoms are extremely severe. There are currently trials underway to find an alternative to HRT for women who've had, or are at risk of, breast cancer.

Dr Barton told me, 'There are a couple of big longitudinal studies going on at the moment, testing the hypothesis that body-identical HRT is breast cancer neutral. The interim results for those studies have been really encouraging, but we don't know for sure. I don't think we'll ever really know for sure, to be honest, because women in their forties, fifties and sixties are the ones using hormone therapy predominantly. And it's women in their forties, fifties and sixties who are also most at risk of getting breast cancer.'

Our breast cells, as with all our cells, are getting older, and that does increase cancer risk. Adding oestrogen and progesterone in the form of hormone therapy can then be an additional breast cancer risk. 'But,' Dr Barton explains, 'from a breast cancer perspective, the biggest risk factors are being overweight and inactive. I find myself saying to patients a lot of the time, "You're taking combined hormones and you're above the age of sixty. So there might be an increased risk of breast cancer. But you're having regular mammograms and you regularly examine your breasts. You've got no family history, or personal history, of breast problems. And by being on HRT we're helping to keep your metabolic health more even and provide you with the capacity you might need to help you sleep better and have more energy to exercise, eat well and make healthy decisions."'

OTHER CAUSES OF INCREASED CANCER RISK

Genetics

Every one of us has genetically predetermined risks in terms of all cancers. They're not necessarily dependent on our parents, although there are some cancers that are strongly inheritable, and there are often other environmental factors at play. Dr Fionnuala Barton explains, 'Our experiences, childhood upbringing, lifestyle choices and environment will all influence how our genes are expressed. There is a lot we cannot reverse or change. We can only really focus on what we have within our power to control to good effect from now and moving forwards.'

Smoking

You don't need me to tell you to quit smoking. You know that, right?

Weight gain

Being overweight is the second biggest cause of cancer in the UK, after smoking. At least one in twenty cancers in the UK (about 22,000 cases) are caused by excess weight. Excess fat cells are inflammatory, which can increase the risk of cancer, and increase levels of growth hormones in the body. These hormones can send signals to cells telling them to divide: if this process goes wrong, it's more likely that a tumour will develop. Post-menopause, fat cells make the weaker form of oestrogen called estrone. This process can make cells in the breast and uterus divide more often, which also increases the risk of a tumour developing.

Alcohol

Drinking increases cancer risk in a way that is dose-dependent, i.e. the more we drink, the greater our risk. A study examining medical records of four million adults with an average age of fifty-four found that giving up drinking has a positive impact on all cancer risk.[122] The highest risks were among people drinking three units a day. Alcohol appears to inhibit the work of natural killer cells within the body that break down cancer cells.

POWER UP: HOW TO REDUCE CANCER RISK

Reducing alcohol intake, not smoking, a healthy diet, exercise and keeping weight under control – as described elsewhere in this book – will all make a difference to cancer risk.

The other element to reducing our cancer risk is being aware of our own bodies, noticing any unexplained symptoms, monitoring our health, going for smears and colon cancer tests when we're asked to. Regular checks of breasts and vulvas are also vital. Here's how to do it.

Vulval check

The vulva is the external parts of female genitalia, not the vagina. To check it, get naked and get in some good light. Use a handheld mirror to check over the vulva, noting any lumps, sores, bumps, tears, white patches, shrinkage of the labia (the inner lips), or changes to the clitoris. How does it feel? How does it look? Any itching? Take photos and keep a record of what you see.

Vulva Cancer Awareness UK has lots of resources on its website, www.lsvcukawareness.co.uk, including information about lichen sclerosus, an itchy condition that can cause patches on vulval skin. It's most common among post-menopausal women and is associated with an increased risk of vulval cancer.

Breast check

We need to check our breasts every month. The first step is to get to know our own breast tissue: what does 'normal' look and feel like? We're much more likely to be able to identify changes if we're starting from a place of knowledge.

There's no right way to check, but the simplest is to use flat fingers and gentle but firm pressure to press on the skin. Feel all the way from your rib cage up towards the breastbone and out to armpits. Note any changes in size, shape and skin texture as well as feeling for lumps. Don't forget your nipples. Try it in front of a mirror, in bed or in the shower. Of course, if you feel anything untoward, contact your doctor.

The charity Coppafeel has more information at coppafeel. org and will send regular 'boob check' reminders if you sign up. I always do my check in the shower on the last day of the month.

Final Thoughts

This book is packed with information, tips and strategies. It's a lot to take on board, I know that. And I had planned to pack even more into this last section, but I think you know enough now. You have all the tools you need to live your own power decade. I don't want to leave you feeling overwhelmed by feeling you 'should' do more. It's time to write your own ending.

If I could say only one thing to you, it would be 'prioritise your own health'. Do whatever it takes to be able to work on your mindset, your meals and your movement. It might be one tiny action, but if you're able to put yourself – and your needs – first, it will be a huge leap. Go back to the 'How do you feel right now?' questionnaire in Section 1 (page 39). Look at it again and see what you've learned as you've read this book, and what you now want to change. Each step you take will move you towards healthy ageing and a vibrant future.

Dr Fionnuala Barton told me, 'This may be an unpopular opinion, but we need to be comfortable with taking responsibility for avoiding reaching a crisis point where we need "fixing" and be empowered in the knowledge that we are all capable of profoundly improving our current health, future health and longevity.'

What are you capable of? Take the time to assess who you are and what you need now you're post-menopausal. Menopause is a time of transformation, when you can be who you want to be. Remember that you are biologically designed to be powerful at this stage of your life. It's hardwired into your DNA: embrace this incredible opportunity to power up your health.

– Susan

www.susansaundershealth.com
@susansaundershealth

Power Women: Rachel Lankester

Rachel, 56, helps women to feel empowered to embrace what may be the best stage of their lives yet. She's founder of the Magnificent Midlife platform and podcast, and author of the brilliant book of the same name. When I spoke to Rachel, she'd just moved back temporarily to her childhood home to take care of her mum, who'd broken her hip. It's a telling example of the complexities of the power decade, building a fantastic new life but also having to deal with responsibility, caring and momentous change.

I asked Rachel how she was navigating her way through life post-menopause. She told me, 'I do think this is the time where we have to look inside and deal with unresolved issues, because we're saying goodbye to one side of our lives and the way we used to be. We have to say goodbye to certain things that we aren't any more and we have to get the balance right between acceptance and still pushing forward to do what we want to do. We have this innate ability within ourselves to be everything we need to be. We are different now, and we can be powerful.'

Rachel experienced her own menopause in her early forties, and feels declining oestrogen levels give us freedom. 'I call oestrogen the biddable hormone, and once it's diminished we have the opportunity to become strong, powerful older women. I think one of the most magnificent things about going through menopause is that we can start putting ourselves first and become who we were always meant to be. This is us, without the impact of oestrogen and our cycles. This can be our most authentic selves. Post-menopause can be so powerful and I want women to realise that, so they don't have to cling on to who they were, but can embrace who they're becoming. Because the world needs us, the world needs feminine energy with extra post-menopausal fire.'

Rachel is very aware of the toll stress takes on our health. 'Our body has a back-up plan to produce oestrogen post-menopause in our adrenal glands. But because there's so much more stress in modern life and so many toxins in our environment, and because we don't always look after ourselves, the body isn't able to prioritise that oestrogen production. I believe that the menopause experience is much worse now because of our diet, stress, ageism and how we feel about getting older. If we're positive about menopause, we're going to have a more positive experience of it. If we're stressed about it, if we're hanging on for dear life because we see menopause as a failure and a deficiency, then we're not going to embrace it. We're not going to feel its power and its strength.

'I'm stronger, I'm more confident, I'm more focused. And I'm also obviously in the second half of life. That really focusses the mind; the clock is ticking. And I think menopausal rage is amazing: we're scared of it because we're not supposed to get angry.

We're supposed to be nice, biddable, "good" women and we don't know what to do with this anger. But that doesn't mean the anger is wrong. And I have found that incredibly empowering. I left my job and started my next chapter because I didn't want to waste any more time doing stuff that didn't make me excited or happy.

'I wanted to set up my business because I was so annoyed about the negative narratives surrounding menopause and women ageing. I was so frustrated that women were floundering, as I had, because they didn't have the information they needed. So now I have a portfolio career: I still do a bit of my previous role in financial communications, I have my magazine *The Mutton Club*, I've got the book, the podcast and I mentor midlife women as well. I make less money than when I worked full-time in communications, but I'm so much happier, and I never get bored of this.'

I asked Rachel what would she say to a woman who wants to create a magnificent, powerful, post-menopausal life? 'It starts with self-belief. You have to believe that you can do it, and that you're meant to do it. Don't listen to people who tell you you can't do it, or you're too old. You're never too old and it's never too late. I think you have to believe in yourself and believe that what you have is what the world needs. We desperately need older women to step forward with all their knowledge and experience. It's just going to waste a lot of the time. We can contribute to the invisibility of older women by shrinking back, by accepting what society expects of us. Whereas we can turn that on its head completely and say, "If there were no limitations on me whatsoever, what do I want to do with the rest of my life?"'

Find Rachel at magnificentmidlife.com and @magnificentmidlife on Instagram and Facebook.

Power Women: Tracy Acock

Tracy, 63, a former cancer-specialist nurse, is a positive life coach and wellbeing practitioner. She works with women in midlife and beyond to help them live a happy, healthy and confident life through her beautifully named platform, The Wellbeing Wisdom Club. Her own wisdom was hard-won through a menopausal rollercoaster that saw her give up the job she loved, then return to nursing before finding new meaning and purpose with coaching. Living in Cornwall, she's a joyous winter wild swimmer.

Tracy found herself struggling to cope with her senior role in breast cancer nursing in her late forties. 'I thought I was stressed because I couldn't handle things in the same way that I used to. I later found out it was perimenopause, but I had no idea at the time. I worked in women's health, and I genuinely didn't know that the heavy bleeding, the anxiety and the loss of confidence were menopausal symptoms. When I turned fifty, my dad died of cancer, I was working in cancer care, and it was all too much. I had to walk away.'

A combination of HRT and good lifestyle habits helped her get back on track. 'What I learned was that it's lifestyle and mindset and taking small steps towards routines that can make a difference.

I went back to cancer care and the biggest job of my career at fifty-five. It's never too late! I set up a Macmillan-funded service for women with secondary breast cancer in three hospitals. It's such a source of pride that I was able to do that.

'Working in the world of cancer changed me. You realise you only get one life. I've definitely been driven in some subconscious way to want to make the most of my health and being here on this planet. That's a driver for me. I've embedded routines that get me moving and get me out in the morning. It might only take five minutes, but it's a start. I've found meditation, which calms the mind, and I have a gratitude practice where I write down three things I'm grateful for each day. Health is always at the centre of that. It doesn't have to be complicated. I've learned that if we can notice how we speak to ourselves, be our biggest cheerleader rather than be mean, we can be our own chief supporter.'

Tracy believes mindset is key to how we approach life in our fifties and sixties. 'There's no timeline to your own life; what is meant for you will come your way. And if it's not meant for you, accept and let go. We're not looking back in the rear-view mirror of life, we're looking forward. It's never too late for self-growth: you can learn more about yourself. You can start a new career, you can pick up a kettlebell for the first time, it's limitless.'

Building routines has been central to keeping Tracy on track. 'In all the changes I've made, there's been some sort of routine in there, there's been something to get up for. It needn't be complicated. I swim almost every day. It's a challenge. But as you build up your routines and your rituals, they become part of you. Find the thing you love and do that every day!'

Tracy finds that confidence post-menopause doesn't always come naturally to her clients. 'Women come to me because they're still wondering where that confidence is. Some feel a sense of lacking, and need help to bring abundance back into their lives. Confidence is like a muscle: the more you use it, the more it grows. The trouble is that, if you're feeling really, really low, it doesn't just happen naturally, so you need a bit of guidance and encouragement.'

Find Tracy at wellbeingwisdomclub.com and @thewellbeingwisdomclub on Instagram.

Acknowledgements

So many incredible women contributed to this book, particularly those who inspired its genesis: my clients, colleagues and friends, plus the brilliant Age-Well Project community and my co-author there, Annabel Streets. All, in different ways, articulated the need for a book that would help post-menopausal women support their health while celebrating how much they'd achieved. I hope this book serves that need.

I'm particularly indebted to Doctors Juliet Balfour, Fionnuala Barton and Carys Sonnenberg, who gave so generously of their time and expertise. Deep gratitude, too, to all the experts and Power Women who contributed so enthusiastically to this book: Meera Bhogal, Jackie Lynch, Christien Bird, Jacqueline Hooton, Dr Lucy Ryan, Rebekah Rotstein, Lee Pycroft, Fay Reid, Jo McEwen and Ann Stephens, Jo Moseley, Kanan Thakerar, Karen Arthur, Rachel Lankester and Tracy Acock.

Many, many women globally have worked tirelessly to put menopause and female reproductive health on the political and medical agenda. There is still more work to be done before all women have access to the menopause support they need. I am indebted to the women who've shouted loud and long about this: without them I would not have been able to get a book published with 'menopause' in the title.

I've referenced multiple academic studies throughout the book, and read many (many) more while writing. My thanks to the researchers who delve deep into the workings of the human body and brain to increase our understanding and improve our health.

Thank you to my agent Rachel Mills, who inspired me to turn the spark of an idea into a book proposal, and to Lindsey Evans at Headline, who saw the potential in that spark on a Zoom call deep in the winter lockdown of 2021. And thank you, both, for your patience while I grappled long and hard to transform that spark into an actual book.

Wider thanks to the teams at Rachel Mills Literary and Headline, particularly Lindsay Davies for her elegant copy editing, Kate Miles for answering my many questions, Louise Rothwell for Production, and Rosie Margesson for Publicity.

Finally, of course, thank you to my fabulous husband and daughters, who supply the power for my own power decade.

Resources

Many of the doctors, health professionals and writers below have a book, socials, a website and a podcast . . . so I've listed websites and Instagram as a starting point, and you can pick and choose how you access the information they share from there. And you can find me at www.susansaundershealth.com and @susansaundershealth on Instagram and Facebook. Come and say hello!

The doctors I interviewed for this book:

Dr Juliet Balfour:
www.wellsmenopauseclinic.co.uk @menopausehealth

Dr Fionnuala Barton:
www.themenopausemedic.com @themenopausemedic

Dr Carys Sonnenberg:
www.rowenahealth.co.uk @drcaryssonnenberg

Other experts I interviewed:

Meera Bhogal:
www.meerabhogal.com @meerabhogal

Jackie Lynch:
www.well-well-well.co.uk @wellwellwelluk

Jacqueline Hooton:
www.hergardengym.co.uk @hergardengym

Christien Bird:
www.whitehartclinic.co.uk @christienbirdphysio

Dr Lucy Ryan:
www.lucyryan.co.uk

Rebekah Rotstein:
www.buff-bones.com @rebekahrotstein

Lee Pycroft:
www.leepycroft.co.uk @leepycroft

The Power Women:

Fay Reid:
www.fayreid.com @9to5menopause

Jacqueline Hooton:
www.hergardengym.co.uk @hergardengym

Jo McEwan and Ann Stephens:
www.positivepause.co.uk @positivepauseuk
www.menopausemovement.co @menopausemovement

Jo Moseley:
www.jomoseley.com @jomoseley

Kanan Thakerar:
www.kananyogabliss.com @kananyogabliss

Karen Arthur:
www.thekarenarthur.com @thekarenarthur
@menopausewhilstblack

Rachel Lankester:
www.magnificentmidlife.com @magnificentmidlife

Tracy Acock:
www.wellbeingwisdomclub.com @thewellbeingwisdomclub

If you're struggling with menopausal symptoms, these experts are brilliant:

Louise Newson:
www.newsonhealth.co.uk @menopause_doctor
and the Balance app

Diane Danzebrink:
www.menopausesupport.co.uk @dianedanzebrink

Amanda Thebe:
www.amandathebe.com @amanda.thebe

Dr Annice Mukherjee:
www.hormonewise.co.uk @the.hormone.doc

Dr Shahzadi Harper:
www.theharperclinic.com @drshahzadiharper

Dr Naomi Potter:

www.menopausecare.co.uk @dr_naomipotter

The books around my desk . . .

If you could look into my tiny cubbyhole of a study, you'd see stacks of books. These are the volumes which piled up around me as I wrote this book:

Bluming, Dr Avrum, and Tavris, Carol, *Oestrogen Matters* (Piatkus, 2018)

Bredesen, Dr Dale, *The End of Alzheimer's Programme* (Vermilion, 2020)

Briden, Lara, *Hormone Repair Manual* (GreenPeak Publishing, 2021)

Brizendine, Dr Louann, *The Upgrade* (Hay House, 2022)

Fitzgerald, Dr Kara, *Younger You* (Quercus, 2022)

Fogg, Dr B. J., *Tiny Habits* (Virgin Books, 2020)

Lynch, Jackie, *The Happy Menopause* (Watkins Publishing, 2020)

Mattern, Susan P., *The Slow Moon Climbs* (Princeton University Press, 2021)

McCall, Davina, with Potter, Dr Naomi, *Menopausing* (HQ, 2022)

Mosconi, Dr Lisa, *The XX Brain* (Allen & Unwin, 2020)

Muir, Kate, *Everything You Need to Know About the Menopause* (Gallery UK, 2022)

Mukherjee, Dr Annice, *The Complete Guide to Menopause* (Vermilion, 2021)

Newson, Dr Louise, *Menopause* (J. H. Haynes & Co Ltd, 2019)

Saunders, Susan, *The Age-Well Plan* (Piatkus, 2020)

Sinclair, Dr David, *Lifespan* (Thorsons, 2019)

Smith, Dr Julie, *Why Has Nobody Told Me This Before?* (Michael Joseph, 2022)

Streets, Annabel, *52 Ways to Walk* (Bloomsbury, 2022)

Streets, Annabel, and Saunders, Susan, *The Age-Well Project* (Piatkus, 2019)

Podcasts

Magnificent Midlife, Rachel Lankester

Menopause Whilst Black, Karen Arthur

Middling Along, Emma Thomas

On My Last Eggs, Rachel New

Postcards from Midlife, Lorraine Candy and Trish Halpin

The Merry Menopause Bookclub, Jo Fuller

The Rollercoaster Podcast, Lucie Q

The Shift with Sam Baker

Websites

www.lattelounge.co.uk

www.menohealth.co.uk

www.menomademodern.com

www.menopause.org

www.menopausemandate.com

www.noon.org.uk

www.overthebloodymoon.com

www.redschoolonline.net

www.talkingmenopause.co.uk

www.thebms.org.uk

www.themenopausecharity.org

Endnotes

1. https://www.ons.gov.uk/
   peoplepopulationandcommunity/
   birthsdeathsandmarriages/lifeexpectancies/bulletins/nation
   allifetablesunitedkingdom/2018to2020
2. https://www.thelancet.com/action/showPdf?pii=S2213-
   8587%2821%2900269-2
3. https://www.ons.gov.uk/
   peoplepopulationandcommunity/healthandsocialcare/
   causesofdeath/articles/leadingcausesofdeathuk/2001to2018
   #uk-leading-causes-of-death-for-all-ages
4. https://www.thelancet.com/journals/landia/article/
   PIIS2213-8587(22)00142-5/fulltext
5. https://jamanetwork.com/journals/jamainternalmedicine/
   fullarticle/2110996
6. https://www.nhs.uk/conditions/menopause/
7. https://www.nhs.uk/conditions/menopause/
8. https://www.nhs.uk/conditions/hysterectomy/
9. https://thebms.org.uk/wp-content/uploads/2022/06/
   Optimising-the-menopause-transition-Joint-position-
   statement.pdf

10. https://www.ncbi.nlm.nih.gov/pmc/articles/PMC5192018/

11. https://www.jneurosci.org/content/26/41/10332

12. Mattern, Susan P., *The Slow Moon Climbs: The Science, History and Meaning of Menopause* (Princeton University Press, 2019)

13. https://pubmed.ncbi.nlm.nih.gov/25706184/

14. https://journals.lww.com/menopausejournal/Abstract/2017/06000/Association_between_anxiety_and_severe.9.aspx

15. https://www.thelancet.com/journals/lancet/article/PIIS0140-6736(19)31709-X/fulltext

16. https://www.ncbi.nlm.nih.gov/pmc/articles/PMC8308420/

17. https://www.tandfonline.com/doi/full/10.1080/1028415X.2022.2084125

18. https://jamanetwork.com/journals/jamanetworkopen/fullarticle/2787246

19. https://link.springer.com/article/10.1007/s00125-022-05752-z

20. https://www.ncbi.nlm.nih.gov/pmc/articles/PMC7468963/

21. https://www.ncbi.nlm.nih.gov/pmc/articles/PMC5808339/

22. https://www.frontiersin.org/articles/10.3389/fendo.2022.886824/full

23. https://pubmed.ncbi.nlm.nih.gov/30661407/

24. https://pubmed.ncbi.nlm.nih.gov/23422924/

25. https://www.nature.com/articles/s41586-021-04010-3

26. https://www.cell.com/cell-reports/pdfExtended/S2211-1247(19)30791-0

27. https://pubmed.ncbi.nlm.nih.gov/12468415/

28. https://pubmed.ncbi.nlm.nih.gov/36094529/

29. https://www.ncbi.nlm.nih.gov/pmc/articles/PMC3976276/

30. https://pubmed.ncbi.nlm.nih.gov/26699485/

31. https://iaap-journals.onlinelibrary.wiley.com/doi/full/10.1111/aphw.12140

32. https://www.ncbi.nlm.nih.gov/pmc/articles/PMC3111147/

33. https://www.ncbi.nlm.nih.gov/pmc/articles/PMC4561742/

34. https://journals.lww.com/menopausejournal/Abstract/2020/09000/The_2020_genitourinary_syndrome_of_menopause.5.aspx

35. https://www.sciencedirect.com/science/article/abs/pii/S0022283619302025?via%3Dihub

36. https://pubmed.ncbi.nlm.nih.gov/25104582/

37. https://pubmed.ncbi.nlm.nih.gov/33832645/

38. https://academic.oup.com/ajcn/article/97/5/1092/4577089

39. https://pubmed.ncbi.nlm.nih.gov/31734757/

40. https://pubmed.ncbi.nlm.nih.gov/29619387/

41. https://www.nhs.uk/conditions/post-menopausal-bleeding/

42. https://joe.bioscientifica.com/view/journals/joe/223/2/R9.xml

43. https://pubmed.ncbi.nlm.nih.gov/24987869/

44. https://www.tandfonline.com/doi/full/10.1080/1028415X.2022.2084125

45. https://pubmed.ncbi.nlm.nih.gov/11978279/

46. https://www.frontiersin.org/articles/10.3389/fnagi.2022.912709/full

47. https://www.ncbi.nlm.nih.gov/pmc/articles/PMC3536461/

48. https://onlinelibrary.wiley.com/doi/10.1111/jdv.18071

49. https://www.ncbi.nlm.nih.gov/pmc/articles/PMC8189331/

50. https://www.researchgate.net/publication/11500389_A_randomized_controlled_trial_of_high_dose_ascorbic_acid_for_reduction_of_blood_pressure_cortisol_and_subjective_responses_to_psychological_stress

51. https://pubmed.ncbi.nlm.nih.gov/17013636/

52. https://www.ncbi.nlm.nih.gov/pmc/articles/PMC3122509/

53. https://files.digital.nhs.uk/9D/4195D5/HSE19-Overweight-obesity-rep.pdf

54. https://www.thelancet.com/journals/ebiom/article/PIIS2352-3964(22)00485-6/fulltext

55. https://pubmed.ncbi.nlm.nih.gov/22766891/

56. https://pubmed.ncbi.nlm.nih.gov/34102108/

57. https://www.termedia.pl/Obesity-in-menopause-our-negligence-or-an-unfortunate-inevitability-,4,30164,1,1.html

58. https://onlinelibrary.wiley.com/doi/full/10.1002/oby.21733

59. https://www.gwern.net/docs/genetics/heritable/2004-simonen.pdf

60. https://journals.plos.org/plosone/article?id=10.1371/journal.pone.0267277

61. https://www.nuffieldhealth.com/healthiernation

62. https://pubmed.ncbi.nlm.nih.gov/35933573/

63. https://pubmed.ncbi.nlm.nih.gov/35033227/

64. https://pubmed.ncbi.nlm.nih.gov/26300634/

65. https://link.springer.com/article/10.1007/s40279-022-01649-4

66. https://www.who.int/news-room/fact-sheets/detail/the-top-10-causes-of-death

67. https://www.bhf.org.uk/informationsupport/conditions/heart-attack/women-and-heart-attacks

68. https://www.whijournal.com/article/S1049-3867(15)00103-6/fulltext

69. https://www.thelancet.com/journals/landia/article/PIIS2213-8587(22)00076-6/fulltext

70. https://www.frontiersin.org/articles/10.3389/fragi.2021.727380/full

71. https://www.ahajournals.org/doi/10.1161/CIR.0000000000000912

72. https://www.ncbi.nlm.nih.gov/pmc/articles/PMC8742618/

73. https://www.frontiersin.org/articles/10.3389/fragi.2021.727380/full

74. https://pubmed.ncbi.nlm.nih.gov/27315068/

75. https://www.ncbi.nlm.nih.gov/pmc/articles/PMC4621258/

76. https://pubmed.ncbi.nlm.nih.gov/32138974/

77. https://www.ncbi.nlm.nih.gov/pmc/articles/PMC2856606/

78. https://pubmed.ncbi.nlm.nih.gov/32187130/

79. https://www.thelancet.com/journals/lancet/article/PIIS0140-6736(16)31714-7/fulltext

80. https://pubmed.ncbi.nlm.nih.gov/26213688/

81. https://academic.oup.com/eurheartj/article/43/30/2867/6612684?login=false

82. https://www.ncbi.nlm.nih.gov/pmc/articles/PMC4425174/

83. https://www.ncbi.nlm.nih.gov/pmc/articles/PMC3735277/

84. https://journals.lww.com/menopausejournal/Citation/2022/01000/Association_between_eating_alone_and.14.aspx

85. https://www.ahajournals.org/doi/10.1161/JAHA.120.017511

86. https://www.alphagalileo.org/en-gb/Item-Display/ItemId/170906?returnurl=https://www.alphagalileo.org/en-gb/Item-Display/ItemId/170906

87. https://www.eurekalert.org/news-releases/587537

88. https://academic.oup.com/eurheartj/article-abstract/43/18/1731/6448753

89. https://pubmed.ncbi.nlm.nih.gov/35785965/

90. https://pubmed.ncbi.nlm.nih.gov/33251828/

92. https://pubmed.ncbi.nlm.nih.gov/27028912/#affiliation-1

93. https://www.sciencedirect.com/science/article/pii/S0049384819304487

94. https://www.nhs.uk/conditions/osteoporosis/causes/

95. https://www.ncbi.nlm.nih.gov/pmc/articles/PMC5643776/

96. https://www.ncbi.nlm.nih.gov/pmc/articles/PMC3424385/

97. https://pubmed.ncbi.nlm.nih.gov/16758142/

98. https://www.ncbi.nlm.nih.gov/pmc/articles/PMC3953885/

99. https://asbmr.onlinelibrary.wiley.com/doi/10.1002/jbmr.3284

100. https://www.ons.gov.uk/peoplepopulationandcommunity/birthsdeathsandmarriages/deaths/bulletins/monthlymortalityanalysisenglandandwales/july2022#death-registrations-and-the-overall-mortality-rate-for-july-2022

101. https://www.thelancet.com/article/S0140-6736(20)30367-6/fulltext

102. https://www.lisamosconi.com/projects

103. http://www.nature.com/articles/s41598-021-90084-y

104. https://www.nature.com/articles/s41598-021-90084-y

105. https://www.ncbi.nlm.nih.gov/pmc/articles/PMC4490700/#!po=1.11111

106. https://www.ncbi.nlm.nih.gov/pmc/articles/PMC6254097/

107. https://content.iospress.com/articles/journal-of-alzheimers disease/jad180164

108. https://journals.plos.org/plosone/article?id=10.1371/journal.pone.0066069

109. https://www.frontiersin.org/articles/10.3389/fnins.2018.00336/full

110. https://pubmed.ncbi.nlm.nih.gov/34027024/

111. https://journals.plos.org/plosone/article?id=10.1371/journal.pone.0235174#sec024

112. https://www.maturitas.org/article/S0378-5122(06)00375-6/fulltext

113. https://jneuroinflammation.biomedcentral.com/articles/10.1186/s12974-020-01998-9

114. https://www.ncbi.nlm.nih.gov/pmc/articles/PMC4738080/

115. https://www.jneurosci.org/content/42/2/288

116. https://www.ncbi.nlm.nih.gov/pmc/articles/PMC6501433/

117. https://www.ncbi.nlm.nih.gov/pmc/articles/PMC6426003/

118. https://www.apa.org/pubs/journals/releases/emo-emo0000343.pdf

119. https://neurology.org/content/97/24/e2381

120. https://pubmed.ncbi.nlm.nih.gov/34311679/

121. https://www.cell.com/cell/fulltext/S0092-8674(19)30850-5

122. https://www.sciencedirect.com/science/article/abs/pii/S0889159116305645

123. https://jamanetwork.com/journals/jamanetworkopen/fullarticle/2795595#:~:text=Conclusions%20and%20Relevance%20Results%20of,alcohol%2Drelated%20and%20all%20cancers.

Index

Index

Index

Index